Ophthalmic Lenses

Ophthalmic Lenses

Second Edition

Ajay Kumar Bhootra
B Optom DOS FAO FOAI FCLI
ICLEP FIACLE (Australia)
Diploma in Sportvision (UK)

Ex-CEO and Dean
Krishnalaya School of Optometry
Kolkata, West Bengal, India

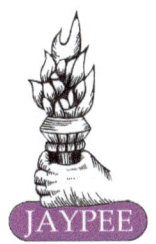

JAYPEE BROTHERS MEDICAL PUBLISHERS
The Health Sciences Publisher
New Delhi | London

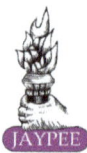 **Jaypee Brothers Medical Publishers (P) Ltd**

Headquarters

Jaypee Brothers Medical Publishers (P) Ltd
EMCA House, 23/23-B
Ansari Road, Daryaganj
New Delhi 110 002, India
Landline: +91-11-23272143, +91-11-23272703
+91-11-23282021, +91-11-23245672
Email: jaypee@jaypeebrothers.com

Corporate Office

Jaypee Brothers Medical Publishers (P) Ltd
4838/24, Ansari Road, Daryaganj
New Delhi 110 002, India
Phone: +91-11-43574357
Fax: +91-11-43574314
Email: jaypee@jaypeebrothers.com

Overseas Office

J.P. Medical Ltd
83 Victoria Street, London
SW1H 0HW (UK)
Phone: +44 20 3170 8910
Fax: +44 (0)20 3008 6180
Email: info@jpmedpub.com

Website: www.jaypeebrothers.com
Website: www.jaypeedigital.com

© 2022, Jaypee Brothers Medical Publishers

The views and opinions expressed in this book are solely those of the original contributor(s)/ author(s) and do not necessarily represent those of editor(s) of the book.

All rights reserved. No part of this publication may be reproduced, stored or transmitted in any form or by any means, electronic, mechanical, photocopying, recording or otherwise, without the prior permission in writing of the publishers.

All brand names and product names used in this book are trade names, service marks, trademarks or registered trademarks of their respective owners. The publisher is not associated with any product or vendor mentioned in this book.

Medical knowledge and practice change constantly. This book is designed to provide accurate, authoritative information about the subject matter in question. However, readers are advised to check the most current information available on procedures included and check information from the manufacturer of each product to be administered, to verify the recommended dose, formula, method and duration of administration, adverse effects and contraindications. It is the responsibility of the practitioner to take all appropriate safety precautions. Neither the publisher nor the author(s)/editor(s) assume any liability for any injury and/or damage to persons or property arising from or related to use of material in this book.

This book is sold on the understanding that the publisher is not engaged in providing professional medical services. If such advice or services are required, the services of a competent medical professional should be sought.

Every effort has been made where necessary to contact holders of copyright to obtain permission to reproduce copyright material. If any have been inadvertently overlooked, the publisher will be pleased to make the necessary arrangements at the first opportunity. The **CD/DVD-ROM** (if any) provided in the sealed envelope with this book is complimentary and free of cost. **Not meant for sale.**

Inquiries for bulk sales may be solicited at: jaypee@jaypeebrothers.com

Ophthalmic Lenses

First Edition: 2009

Second Edition: **2022**

ISBN: 978-93-90595-40-2

Printed at

Dedicated to

My parents Mr Ashok Kumar Bhootra and
Mrs Kamalesh Bhootra
My late grandparents Sri Bhagwan Das Bhootra and
Smt Shanti Devi Bhootra
My beloved uncle Sri Radhe Shyam Bhootra
Who have always been appreciating all my books

A
Tribute
to
Late Krishna Kumar Binani

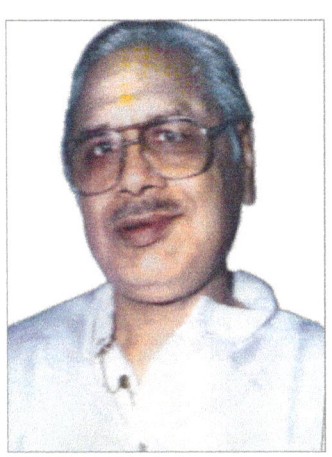

A passionate Samaritan,
An astute industry representative,
A foresighted businessman,
A great connoisseur of literature,
A devoted social worker,
A great family person,
A dutiful husband,
A caring father,
A fatherly employer,
My biggest inspiration and mentor.

Ajay Kumar Bhootra

Preface to the Second Edition

The year 2020 has changed everything. Every year typically has a few defining moments, but the year 2020 have contained so many world-changing and paradigm-shifting developments that it's getting hard to believe we're not in a simulation that's running every possible scenario at once.

The COVID-19 pandemic dominated the year, raging the world across. We had never seen a catastrophe like this. Lot of people died from COVID-19. Markets across the globe shuddered and crashed. Worldwide lockdowns and restrictions incarcerated people to their home. Working from home has been more difficult than convenient for most.

Everyone wanted normalcy, but normalcy was out of sight; face masks, social distancing, and working from home became the "new normal". The crisis forced people to confront a new world that is ever changing, unpredictable and uncontrollable. Fear, frustration, and anxiety levels touched their peak.

The current situation - whether we like it or not, is here to stay for a while. People have little control over it or its resolution. Though we may mitigate the health risks of the virus in the near future, its financial implications will surely last for years. So, what matters is how we choose to respond to it. There seems to be only two options—either embrace the COVID -19 crisis or become victim of it.

Eckhart Tolle, the famous spiritual teacher and bestselling author, has said, "Accept, then act. Whatever the present moment contains, embrace it as if you had chosen it. This will miraculously change your life."

While what Tolle says holds true, it is easier said than done. Even if we accept a crisis like COVID-19 as a part of our everyday lives, we are far from living only in the present. Our minds, involuntarily get cluttered with the broken memories of past and fears of future, naively believing that everything would be perfect again.

For me, fortunately, the crisis was only at the back of my mind, as I was focused on working upon the second edition of *Ophthalmic Lenses* and *Dispensing Optics*. Dispensing optics is one of the most fascinating branches of optometry. Ironically, many optometry students today look upon dispensing optics with a deep-seated feeling of aversion. But it is the most elastic and satisfying subject among all the subjects covered under the optometry discipline.

Most optometrists spend time on prescription of spectacles and contact lens fitting. They are comfortable with this, as it allows them to work as the clinician. But dispensing optics has a broader scope. It allows optometrists to look beyond the boundaries of clinical practice, and opens the door for them to work at the management level. In a world where competition is cut-throat and excellence is indispensable, it is important for optometrists to consider this lucrative and rewarding subject.

The second edition of *Ophthalmic Lenses* is designed to be a helpful resource for acquiring practical knowledge pertaining to ophthalmic lenses, their optics and applications. This edition is more organized and rich, as far as resource material is concerned. The revisions made in this edition include:
- Multiple Choice Questions at the end of each chapter, to better aid students in their learning process
- A new chapter, titled Specialty Lenses
- Updation and elaboration of existing chapters
- Graphs and flowcharts to make the book reader friendly.

The ophthalmic lens technology has witnessed several new developments, in the last few years. More complex and technologically driven lenses have been introduced. Personalization and customization of lenses are at the forefront of current research. These new lenses cater to very specific needs, and they need to be dispensed with additional dispensing measurements. For example, standard progressive addition lenses are purchased for their functional use, whereas high value progressive addition lenses are sought for their value additions.

Dispensing and selling such lenses requires worked skills. An interrogative discussion on visual needs will create a strong foundation, a correct solution in the form of ophthalmic lens will motivate and arouse confidence in the patient, and a technologically driven consultation will ultimately lead to patient satisfaction. The straight forward implication is that now it is possible to specialize in ophthalmic lens and its technologies alone.

As a parting note, I wish to explicitly state that my core objective behind this edition was to simplify the content, and organize it most appropriately, such that it serves as a go-to reference for ophthalmic lenses. In pursuit of this objective, I request all readers to share with me their valued feedback on my email – stplajay@gmail.com. I'll be delighted to read your comments.

Wishing you a happy and resourceful reading!

Ajay Kumar Bhootra

Preface to the First Edition

As we travel across the world, we see that numerous countries are still missing out on developments. We are fortunate to have almost all the latest developments in the field of ophthalmic lenses. The availability of wide range in the material and design of ophthalmic lenses has made it indispensable to understand the principles of optics behind them to understand their use and practical application. In developed countries, the newer developments in the lens design and material are immediately accepted irrespective of their cost and necessity. This kind of "ready to accept new development" approach is generally not seen in the countries which are on the brink of developments. In those places, the availability of wide range of products creates a typical situation for low income group who look for best at most economical cost. They need to be understood that technological developments are meant to cater to the increasing complexities of life and ever changing lifestyle. And products developed after extensive research and studies also carry the cost of research involved in it. This necessitates the need for detailed information about their technology and application.

Lots of new ophthalmic lenses have been introduced, but unfortunately there is a dearth of good books on this subject. This book is an effort to fill this gap. The need for a book that describes the choice of ophthalmic lenses has been already seen by the kind of acceptance given to author's first book Optician's Guide. But the information presented in this book is designed to provide comprehensive details about the ophthalmic lenses and their dispensing tips. Most of the information will replicate my 22 years of experience in the field of optical dispensing and will be helpful to the students of optometry. In addition, this book may also be of great help to ophthalmologists, opticians, ophthalmic lens manufacturers and all those who would like to excel in the field of optical dispensing.

Finally, it is hoped that the readers of this book will enjoy its simplicity and appreciate its organized presentation.

Ajay Kumar Bhootra

Acknowledgments

Essilor is the world's leading ophthalmic lens manufacturer and distributor. Year after year, Essilor continues to live out its corporate mission—"Helping the world see better by providing excellent vision through premium products and services". Technological advancements and exclusive training programs are the main cornerstone of their every product launch.

Essilor continues to bring innovation to life through research, advances in lens technology, and educational services to the eye care professionals. These three components set Essilor apart from its competitors and characterize Essilor as the world leader in ophthalmic optics. To me, Essilor has always been very humble and kind in sending me information and new ideas on ophthalmic lenses and allied services. Even this book also features lots of pictures, graphical representations and ideas supplied by them.

I firmly accept that I could not have completed this book without Essilor's support. Many thanks to Mr K Sugavanam, General Manager, Essilor Brand who has been so much cooperative to me.

I cannot end without acknowledging the support of Mr Chakravarthy, National Sales Manager, Beauty Glass, Essilor. I am highly indebted to them and the entire team of Essilor for their wholehearted support to me. Without their support, it would have been very difficult for me to transform the idea into a book.

Contents

1. **Basic Optical Principle**   1
   - Laws of Reflection *1*
   - Laws of Refraction *1*
   - Vergence *3*
   - Surface Power and Surface Curvature of Lens *3*
   - Focal Power *5*
   - Thin Lens Power *6*
   - Effect of Thickness on Lens Power *7*
   - Sign Convention *7*
   - Multiple Choice Questions *8*

2. **Ophthalmic Lens Material and Design**   9
   - Glass Material *9*
   - Resin Material *11*
   - Properties of Ophthalmic Lenses *12*
   - Curve Variation Factor *18*
   - Ophthalmic Lens Design *19*
   - Multiple Choice Questions *29*

3. **Spherical Lenses**   31
   - Dioptric Power of Lenses, Vergence *36*
   - Spherical Lens Decentration and Prism Power *36*
   - Detection of Spherical Lens *37*
   - Multiple Choice Questions *39*

4. **Astigmatic Lenses**   41
   - Cylinder Lenses *41*
   - Notation for Cylinder Lenses and Orientation of Axis *42*
   - Toric Lenses *44*
   - Detection of Cylindrical Lens *46*
   - Multiple Choice Questions *49*

5. **Prisms**   50
   - Characteristics of Prism *52*
   - Deviation Produced by Prism *52*
   - Prentice Rule *53*
   - Prism Orientation *53*
   - Splitting or Dividing Prism *54*

- Types of Prism 55
- Uses of Prism 57
- Fresnel Prism 58
- Compounding and Resolving Prisms 58
- Prism and Lens Decentration 61
- Detection of Prism in an Optical Lens 62
- Summary 63
- Multiple Choice Questions 63

6. Lens Aberrations 65

- Chromatic Aberration 66
- Spherical Aberration 67
- Off-axis Astigmatism 69
- Coma 70
- Curvature of Field 70
- Distortion 71
- Multiple Choice Questions 73

7. Tinted Lens 75

- The Electromagnetic Spectrum 75
- Effect of Radiant Energy on the Ocular Tissues 76
- Absorption Characteristics of Conventional Crown Glass 78
- Filter Lenses 78
- Methods of Lens Tinting 82
- Photochromic Lenses 85
- Factors Affecting Photochromatism 85
- Tint Options in Photochromic Lenses 86
- Resin Photochromic Lens 87
- Dispensing Tips for Photochromatic Lenses 88
- Polaroid Lenses 88
- Application of Polarized Lenses 90
- Advantages of Polaroid Lenses 90
- Tints vs Polarized Lenses 90
- Dispensing Tips for Polaroid Lenses 91
- Prescribing Tints 91
- Blue Light and Blue Cut Lenses 93
- Multiple Choice Questions 95

8. Anti-reflection Coated Lens 97

- The Reflection of Light 97
- Principle of Anti-reflection Coating 98
- Single Layer Anti-reflection Coating 100
- Multilayer Anti-reflection Coating 101

- Advantages of Anti-reflection Coating *103*
- Anti-reflection Coating of Pretinted Lenses *104*
- Dispensing Tips *104*
- Technology for Applying Anti-reflection Coating *105*
- Multiple Choice Questions *106*

9. Aspheric Lenses   108

- Why Aspheric? *110*
- Aspheric Lens Design *110*
- Measuring an Aspheric Surface *114*
- Prism in Aspheric Lenses *114*
- Aspheric Lenses for Aphakic Patients *115*
- Checking Lens Power in Aspheric Lens *117*
- Dispensing Tips *117*
- Multiple Choice Questions *118*

10. Bifocal Lenses   120

- Types of Bifocal Lenses *121*
- Bifocal Segment Shapes *126*
- Optical Characteristics of Bifocal Lenses *130*
- Prism Controlled Bifocals *138*
- Invisible Bifocals *142*
- Bifocal Dispensing *142*
- Verification of Segment Height *147*
- Multiple Choice Questions *148*

11. Progressive Addition Lenses   149

- Distance *151*
- Near *151*
- Intermediate *151*
- Basic Design Difference between Progressive, Single Vision, Bifocal and Trifocal Lenses *151*
- Advantages of Progressive Addition Lenses *153*
- Progressive Addition Lens Markings *156*
- Progressive Addition Lens Optical Design *157*
- Minkwitz Rule *160*
- Progressive Addition Lens Designs *160*
- Optical Description of Progressive Addition Lens *163*
- Designing Progressive Addition Lens *169*
- Prism Thinning *172*
- Limitation of Conventional Progressive Addition Lenses *174*
- Restoration of Progressive Addition Lens Markings *175*
- Generating Progressive Power Surface *177*

- Evolution of Progressive Addition Lens *180*
- Current Progressive Lens Design Development *184*
- Who is Suitable for Progressive Addition Lenses? *188*
- Ideal Frame Selection for Progressive Addition Lens *189*
- Dispensing Progressive Addition Lenses *191*
- Multiple Choice Questions *196*

12. Safety Lenses   198

- Lens Materials *200*
- Testing Procedure for Safety Lenses *206*
- Types of Lens Housing *209*
- Regulations and Standards Relating to Eye Protection *210*
- Multiple Choice Questions *212*

13. Surface Treatments   213

- Hard Coating *213*
- Hydrophobic Coating *214*
- Anti-fog Coating *215*
- Anti-mist Coating *216*
- Toughening Glass Lenses *216*
- Surface Tinting of Lenses *217*
- Multiple Choice Questions *218*

14. Sports Lenses   219

- Horizontal Inclination *222*
- Features of Sport Lenses *226*
- Tints and Colors in Sports Lenses *227*
- Presbyopia and Sports Lens *230*
- Summary *231*
- Multiple Choice Questions *231*

15. Specialty Lenses   233

- Iseikonic Lenses *233*
- Regressive Lenses *233*
- Adaptive Lenses *234*
- Anti-fatigue Lens *234*
- Atoric Lenses *235*
- Summary *236*
- Multiple Choice Questions *236*

Bibliography   *237*

Index   *239*

Chapter 1

Basic Optical Principle

An ophthalmic lens is an optical medium that is bound by two polished surfaces, at least one of which must be curved. The curvature may be spherical, toroidal or aspherical. Ophthalmic lens theory is based upon the basic laws of Geometric Optics. The ophthalmic lenses are used to alter the vergence of rays of light and are used to correct some errors of the eyes. For theoretical calculations on ophthalmic lenses, light is assumed to travel in straight lines and that the incident light travels from left to right. It meets a surface that separates two media. What happens to the light, then, depends upon the nature of the surface and the two media on either side. In this chapter, we will consider these fundamental laws of physics and how they relate to the theory of spectacle lenses.

LAWS OF REFLECTION

Light travels in straight line until it meets a surface that separates the two media. When light meets the surface, its behavior depends on the nature of the surface and the two media on either side. Light may be absorbed by the new medium, or transmitted onwards through it, or it may bounce back into the first medium. The bouncing back of light into the incident ray medium is called Reflection of light. The light may reflect specularly if the surface is acting as true mirror or it may reflect diffusely, scattering it in all directions if the surface is incompletely polished. In case of specular reflection, the reflected light obeys the laws of reflection, which states that:
- The incident ray, the reflected ray and the normal ray to the reflecting surface—all lie in the same plane.
- The angle of incidence equals the angle of reflection.

It follows from the laws of reflection that, when an object is placed in front of a plane mirror, the image formed by the mirror lies as far behind the mirror surface as the object lies in front. Also the straight line that joins the object and its reflected image is normal to the mirror surface **(Fig. 1.1)**.

LAWS OF REFRACTION

Refraction is defined as the change in direction of light when it passes from one transparent medium into another of different optical density. The incident ray, the refracted ray and the normal—all lies in the same plane. The refracted light undergoes a change in velocity. The ratio of the velocities of light in the

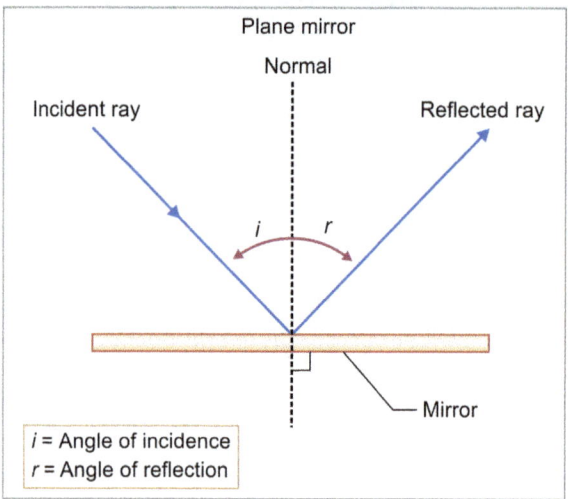

Fig. 1.1: Reflection at the plane surface

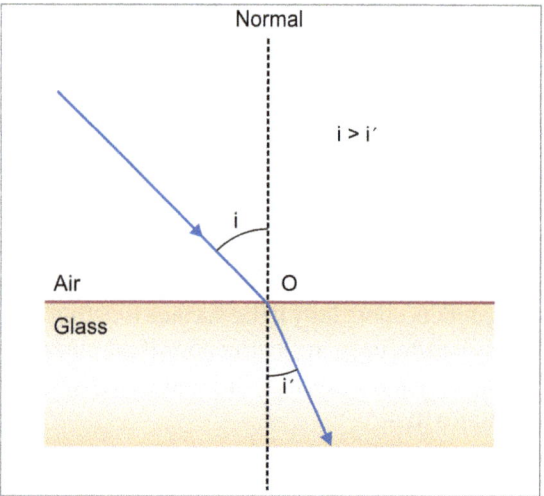

Fig. 1.2: Refraction of light entering an optical dense medium from air

first and second media is called the relative refractive index between the media, which slows with denser medium. The absolute refractive index of a medium "n" is defined as the ratio of the velocity of light in vacuum to the velocity of light in the respective medium:

$$\text{Refractive index (n)} = \frac{\text{Velocity of light in vacuum}}{\text{Velocity of light in the medium}}$$

Figure 1.2 illustrates a ray of light that is incident, in air at point D on the surface of a plane—solid glass block. The refractive index of the first medium (air) is denoted by n and the refractive index of the second medium (glass

block) is denoted by n'. The angle of incidence that the incident ray makes with the normal to the surface at D is denoted by n and the angle of refraction is denoted by n'. The laws of refraction (Snell's law) state that:
- The incident ray, the refracted ray and the normal to the surface at the point of incidence—all lie in one plane.
- The ratio of the angle of incidence, i, to the angle of refraction, i', is constant for any two media.

The most important application of this Snell's law of refraction is to determine the effect of prisms and lenses on the incident light, that is to determine the change in direction and the change in vergence produced by a lens.

■ VERGENCE

Vergence is the term that determines the direction and power of light transmission. It is the wavefront of light of a particular position in a particular time. Vergence can be understood as a measure of the curvature of the optical wavefront, expressed in "diopter". The vergence of light is defined by:

$$V = \frac{n}{L}$$

Where,
n = Refractive index of the material.
L = The distance in accordance with the Cartesian Sign Convention.

For light propagating away from a source, i.e., diverging, the vergence is negative, given by following formula:

$$V = \frac{-n}{L}$$

For light propagating towards a focus, i.e., converging, the vergence is positive, given by following formula:

$$V = \frac{+n}{L}$$

Since the distance L_1 is measured from the wavefront and the light is traveling from left to right, it is a negative distance and the vergence is negative (divergent). L_2 is positive since it is directed to the right from the wavefront (convergent). Parallel light rays are said to have zero vergence. The change in vergence when the light encounters a refracting surface is equal to the power of the surface **(Fig. 1.3)**.

■ SURFACE POWER AND SURFACE CURVATURE OF LENS

The ability of a surface of the lens to alter the vergence of incident light is called its surface power. A lens has two surfaces, either of which may be positive or negative or flat, separated by a thickness of lens material. Each surface of a lens will have a converging or diverging effect of its own which depends upon the radius of curvature of the surface and the refractive index of the material. The

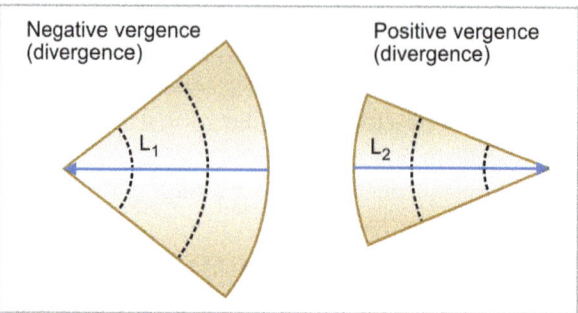

Fig. 1.3: Vergence is measured from the wavefront. Positive is in the direction of light travel

power of each surface contributes to the total focal power of the lens. When the front surface or positive surface is stronger than back surface or negative surface, the lens is generally plus lens and when the back surface or negative surface power is stronger than front surface it is generally a minus lens. And when the front surface power is equal to that of the back surface, the net power of the two surfaces is zero and the lens is usually termed as plano lens.

Surface curvature, on the other hand is the geometrical property of the surface of the lens. In case of simple spherical surface, it depends only on radius of curvature of the surface. Surface curvature is the angle through which the surface turns in unit length of arc. The larger the radius of curvature, the flatter the curvature of the surface and shorter the radius of curvature, the steeper the curvature of the surface. The radius of curvature of a surface is inversely proportional to its surface power which implies steeper surface will produce stronger focal power of the lens than flatter surface.

Figure 1.4 illustrates a cross-sectional view of different curved forms of spherical surface. Spherical surface has uniform curvature in all its zones, whereas, in case of surfaces other than spherical, the curvature varies in different zones and from one meridian to another.

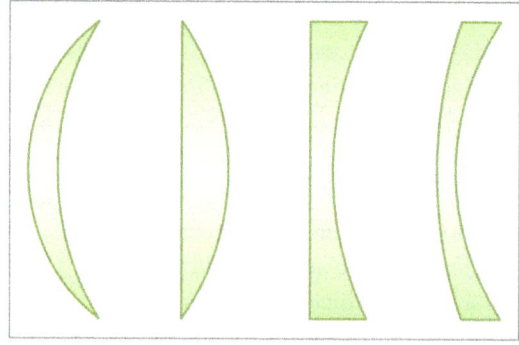

Fig. 1.4: Forms of curvature

The curvature of a spherical surface can be read with a simple instrument called "spherometer", which measures the height of the vertex of the curve above a fixed chord **(Fig. 1.5)**.

The common form of spherometer normally available is the "Optician's lens measure" which is calibrated for a refractive index of 1.523 and gives the diopter power of the surface directly. More accurate version of this simple lens measure is used in surfacing laboratory and is known as "sagometers" **(Fig. 1.6)**.

FOCAL POWER

The total power of a lens to bend light is referred to as its focal power. Units of focal power are expressed as "diopter" and are related to the focal length of the lens. The relationship between focal length and focal power can be expressed by the formula:

$$F = \frac{n}{f}$$

Where, F = Focal power in diopter.
f = Focal length of the lens in metres.
n = Refractive index of the medium in which the light is traveling.

Since the other medium is always air while working with spectacle lenses, the relationship can be simplified to:

$$F = \frac{1}{F}$$

A plus lens has positive focal length as the second principal focus point of plus lens lies to the right of the lens, whereas a minus lens has negative focal length as the second principal focus of minus lens lies to the left of the lens. A lens with zero power whose focal length is infinitely long is denoted by the sign infinity. Such a lens is also known as afocal lens.

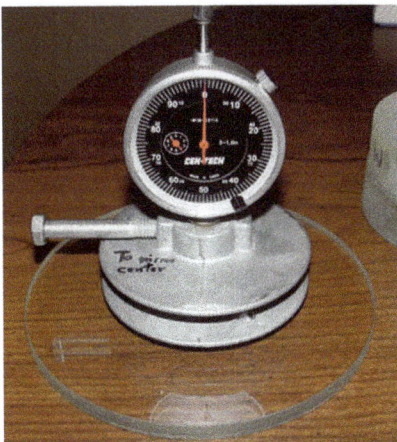

Fig. 1.5: Spherometer

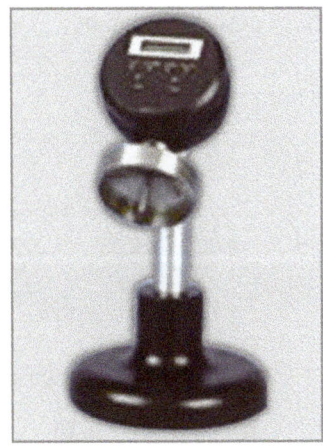

Fig 1.6: Sagometer

Examples:
Focal power of lens that has focal length of – 100 cm
F = 100/f (in cm)
F = 100/–100
F = – 1.00 D

Focal power of lens that has focal length of + 625 mm
F = 1000/f (in mm)
F = 1000/625
F = +1.60 D

THIN LENS POWER

In optical dispensing while calculating the power of the lens, the effect of the lens thickness is ruled out. The total thin lens power of the lens is the sum of its surface powers. For example, if a lens has a front surface power of + 8.00D and back surface power of – 4.00D, then its thin lens power is + 4.00D.

Theoretically, we could make + 4.00D lens in any form as shown in **Figure 1.7** in which the first form has both sides convex surfaces and is known as biconvex lens form. The second form which has one plane surface is known as plano convex lens form. The other forms in the figure, each has one convex surface and one concave surface and are known as curved or meniscus lenses. In practice, modern lenses are curved in form. The surface power of a curved lens may be different at its two principal meridians, in which case the lower numerical surface power is taken as the base curve.

The relationship between the two surface powers F_1 and F_2 and the total thin lens power of the lens F is:

$$F = F_1 + F_2$$

If the refractive index of the lens is denoted by 'n' and radii of curvature of the front and back surfaces are r_1 and r_2 respectively then the individual surface power is given by:

$$F_1 = \frac{n-1}{r_1}$$

$$\text{And, } F_2 = \frac{1-n}{r_2}$$

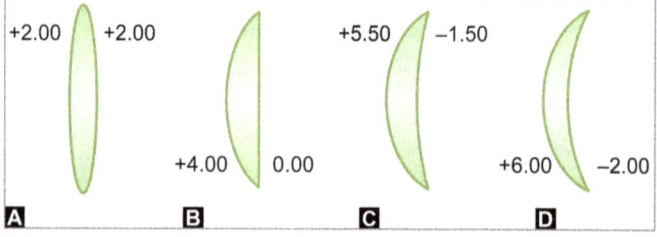

Fig.1.7: Various forms in which + 4.00D lens might be made

These two equations can be combined into the lens maker's equation:
$$F = (n - 1)(1/r_1 - 1/r_2)$$

EFFECT OF THICKNESS ON LENS POWER

When the thickness of the lens is taken into account the actual power of the lens cannot be found from the simple sum of the surface powers, but it can be found by considering the change of vergence that the light undergoes after refraction at one surface and finally at the back surface. In case of a thick lens, the light after refraction from F_1 will have a chance to travel a given distance before reaching F_2 as it continues to travel through the lens thickness, it will have a slightly different vergence from when it left F_1. It is this new vergence that F_2 alters to produce an existing vergence.

SIGN CONVENTION

Light is assumed to be passing from left to right and the measurement taken in the course of light is taken as positive and the measurement taken against the course of light is taken as negative. All distances are measured from the vertex of the lens to the point in question. The sign convention is used to represent whether the corresponding surface is convex or concave **(Fig. 1.8)**. It says that:
- Distances to the left are negative
- Distances to the right are positive
- Distances above the optical axis are positive
- Distances below the optical axis are negative.

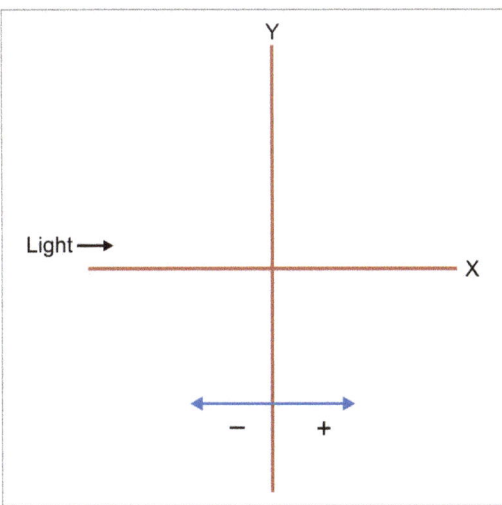

Fig. 1.8: Sign convention

Ophthalmic Lenses

 Multiple Choice Questions (MCQs)

1. Which of the following is correct for reflection of light by smooth surface?
   a. It is called regular reflection
   b. It is called irregular reflection
   c. It is called regular refraction
   d. It is called irregular refraction

2. Which of the following is correct for reflection of light by rough surface?
   a. It is called regular reflection
   b. It is called irregular reflection
   c. It is called regular refraction
   d. It is called irregular refraction

3. When light traveling in a certain medium falls on surface of another medium, a part of it turns back in same medium. What is this phenomenon known as?
   a. Reflection
   b. Refraction
   c. Diffraction
   d. Acoustics

4. The rays of light after reflecting from a rough surface travel in:
   a. Two directions
   b. One direction
   c. Many directions
   d. Directionless

5. According to law of reflection the angle of incidence and angle of reflection are:
   a. Both negative
   b. Unequal
   c. Equal
   d. Opposite

6. Light bending effect as it passes from one transparent material into other material with different refractive index is known as:
   a. Reflection
   b. Diffraction
   c. Refraction
   d. Deflection

7. Focal length of plano lens is:
   a. Infinity
   b. Zero
   c. Negative
   d. None of the above

8. Which of the following is *not* true about surface power of the lens?
   a. Surface power of the lens is the ability of each surface of the lens to alter the vergence of incident light.
   b. The power of each surface of the lens contributes to the total focal power of the lens.
   c. Surface power denotes the geometrical property of the surface of the lens.
   d. None of the above.

Answers

| 1. a | 2. b | 3. a | 4. c | 5. c | 6. c | 7. a | 8. c |

Chapter 2
Ophthalmic Lens Material and Design

Ophthalmic lens materials refer to all materials used during manufacturing of lenses, i.e., all materials entered into the composition of the basic ophthalmic lens. The end result is the new lens material which has specific physical and other properties and specific lens geometry, giving the lens its corrective function—what is referred to as lens design or form. All the ophthalmic lenses currently available in the ophthalmic industry are:
- Glass material
- Resin material

GLASS MATERIAL

The different raw materials are used in a given proportion and composition while manufacturing spectacle lenses so that it can be used to provide its final application, i.e. refracting the rays of light and thereby improving the eyesight. The lenses so made are in the form of semi-finished lens and is not delivered in the form of a ready-to-use lenses. It is, in fact, a molding blank requiring certain finishing operations.

From an optical point of view, a spectacle lens is a medium aimed at directing light along a specific course and therefore, must possess specific optical properties. They are designed for day-to-day use under all conditions. This demands certain mechanical and chemical properties for comfort, safety and long-lasting usage. Lastly, it calls for special manufacturing techniques which make allowance not only for the qualities demanded by spectacle lenses but also for economical production.

The components used for glasses for spectacle lenses are vitrifiable mixture which is put into the melting tank in the form of extremely pure raw materials so as to obtain perfect quality glass. The basic components such as silica and alumina are introduced in the respective forms of iron-free sand and feldspar.

The alkaline oxides (sodium or potassium) are generally added in the form of carbonates or nitrates. Lime and magnesia are sometimes replaced by limestone and dolomite. These basic components are accompanied by numerous other ingredients such as rare earths.

The role of different components is:

Oxides

Oxides are used in the lens compositions primarily into two major categories:

1. *Network formative oxides*: Network formative oxides are used at the base of any composition which could almost form a lens on their own. For example, SiO_2, B_2O_3, P_2O_5.
2. *Modifier oxides:* They are used to modify the basic properties contributed by formative oxides. These may range from viscosity to electric properties or from chemical resistance to coefficient of expansion. For example, K_2O, Na_2O, BaO.

According to composition, some oxides behave either as formatives or as modifiers. They are called intermediary oxides. For example, Al_2O_3, ZnO, TiO_2.

Refiners

Refiners have the basic function of eliminating gaseous inclusions (bubbles) in molten glass. Examples are Antimony Oxide, Alkaline Nitrates.

Colorants

Complete absence of colorants is essential to obtain clear 'white' glass. When added deliberately, they lead to selective absorption for each wavelength in the spectrum and so determine the tints. Example: Cobalt oxide gives rise to blue, Nickel oxides for brown.

The most common glasses currently popular in the industry for ophthalmic lenses are:

Crown

Crown is the most commonly used glasses for spectacle lenses. They belong to the family of the window glasses. They differ essentially through the choice of raw materials and certain additions of ingredients to adjust optical and physical properties. Their composition is characterized by high silica, lime and sodium. The extra white crown is very pure silica-based glass which is extremely transparent. Some crown glasses through the addition of metal oxides like nickel and cobalt show specific tints and absorbent properties.

Photo Chromic Glasses

Owing to the need for the glass to have the special properties of reaction to certain light radiation, the composition is more elaborate. The vitrifiable structure is extremely stable, i.e., a borosilicate with a high boron content to which is added a series of elements introduced to develop microcrystals of silver halide which are responsible for the photochromic phenomenon.

High-Index Glasses

Lead oxide has been traditionally included in the glass composition to produce high index glasses. This produced "flint" glass. Today, for high refractive index glass lead oxide is replaced by titanium oxides, thus preserving high index while reducing glass density. Certain other elements such as niobium, zirconium and strontium are also included for adjusting optical properties.

To obtain an improved range of segment glasses for fused multifocals, lead oxide is replaced by barium oxide.

RESIN MATERIAL

Resin lenses are made up of small molecular units called monomers which link together to form long chain known as polymers and the process of linking the monomers together is known as polymerization. There are two processes to make resin lenses:
1. Thermosetting
2. Thermoplastic.

Thermosetting and thermoplastic differ basically in the lining up of the molecules in their structure **(Figs. 2.1A and B)**. Thermosetting are cross-linked molecular structure, resembles a ladder with extra rungs. They do not melt or flow when heat is applied and makes the material less flexible. Therefore, allows for superior optical processing. CR_{39} is the good example. Most hi-index resin lenses are made by thermosetting process. The monomer liquid is poured into a mould where chemical process of polymerization takes place to form a solid material.

Thermoplastic are not cross-linked molecular structure. Molecular chains are independent of each other, looks like a ladder without rungs. Optically they are not so stable during process. They soften under heat and therefore, good for injection molding process. They are very sensitive to abrasion. Polycarbonates are the good examples.

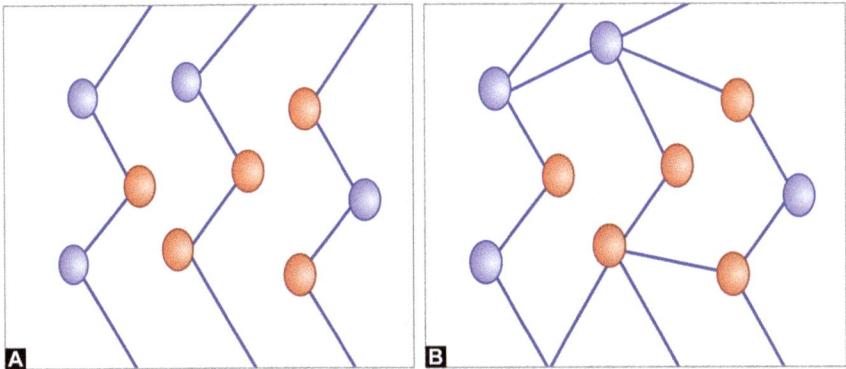

Figs. 2.1A and B: (A) Thermoplastic; (B) Thermosetting

Currently following resin materials are popularly available in the ophthalmic lens industry:

CR_{39}

CR_{39} is thermosetting resin, i.e., in its basic form it is liquid monomer which is hardened by polymerization under the effect of heat and a catalyst. Diethylene glycol bis, better known as CR_{39} is the material most widely used to manufacture currently marketed plastic lens. It was discovered during forties by chemists from the "Columbia Corporation", hence, its name "Columbia Resin # 39". The refractive index of CR_{39} is 1.498, which is close to standard crown glasses, specific gravity is 1.32 gram/cm^3 and abbe value is 58, ensuring low chromatism. The material is highly impact resistant and carries high transparency. Multiple tinting and coating is possible. Only drawback is weak resistant to abrasion.

Polycarbonate

Polycarbonate is a relatively old material, but its use in ophthalmic optics has grown over the past few years. It is linear polymer thermoplastic with an amorphous structure. It is atleast ten times more impact resistant than CR_{39}. A high refractive index of 1.586 makes it comparatively thinner. Specific gravity of 1.20g/cm^3 makes it very light in its weight. The material has efficient protection against ultra violet rays. Abbe value is 30, which is significantly low for good optical performance. The material is very soft in nature and hence prone to scratches. Tinting is relatively difficult with polycarbonate lens material which is usually obtained by impregnating a tintable scratch-resistant coating.

Trivex

Trivex is a partially cross-linked material and uses the best attributes of thermoplastic and thermosetting processes. The result is the superior impact resistance with superior optical performance. The refractive index is 1.53 with a specific gravity of 1.11 gm/cm^3 make the lens thin and light. Probably this is the only lens which is best for rimless frame. Abbe value is 45 and the material has 100% UV protection property. It can be easily tinted and coated with anti-reflection coating.

■ PROPERTIES OF OPHTHALMIC LENSES

When a beam of light falls on a lens surface, some of the light passes through the lens, some of the light is reflected from the lens surface and some of the light is absorbed by the lens material **(Fig. 2.2)**. The measure of the proportion of light reflected from the surface is called reflectance. The measure of proportion of light absorbed is the absorption and the measure of the proportion of light transmitted is the transmittance. Each one is expressed as a fraction of the total quantity of light in the beam. If the intensity of the beam of light is represented

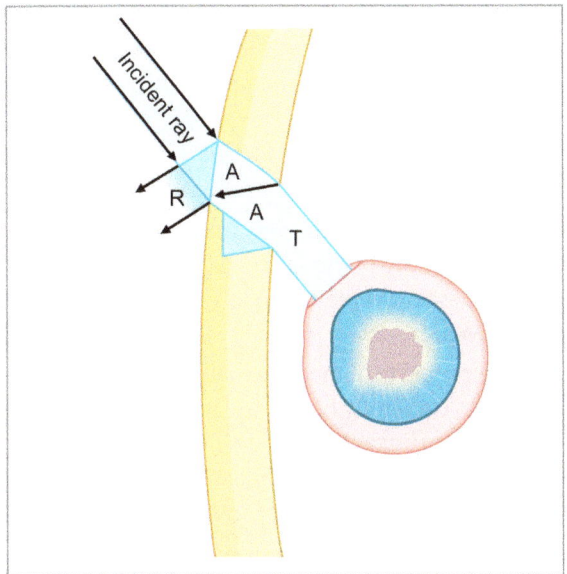

Fig. 2.2: Incident light on an ophthalmic lens

by the number 1, reflectance by R, absorption by A and transmittance by T, the intensity may be expressed as follows:

$$R + A + T = 1$$

The aim of the ophthalmic lenses is to restore clear vision to an ametropic eye by placing a corrective lens between the viewed object and the eye and the dioptric function of the lens depends on the characteristics of the lens material. Extensive knowledge of the properties of these materials is, therefore, needed in the following areas:
- Optical properties
- Mechanical properties
- Electrical properties
- Chemical properties
- Thermal properties

Optical Properties

Optical properties are essential properties of the ophthalmic lens material to calculate the dioptric function and control of optical performance. These properties describe the following features of the lens material:

Abbe Value

Abbe value is the number that is the measure of the degree to which light is dispersed when entering a lens material. Dispersion stands for the amount that the material spreads out the different wavelengths of light passing through it. Abbe number represents the relative degree of distortion generated while looking through off center area of the lens. The lower the abbe number, the greater the dispersion of light, causing the chromatic aberration in the periphery of the lens. The higher the Abbe number, the better the peripheral optics. Abbe number of 60 is considered to have the least chromatic aberrations and abbe number of 30 is for the most chromatic aberrations.

When the wearer moves the eyes away from the center and looks through the periphery of the lens, the prism is created. The amount of prism created together with the dispersion value of the lens material affects the amount of "colour fringes" the wearer sees.

Abbe value is the property of the lens material and can not be affected by any surface technique. Generally higher the index of refraction, the lower the Abbe value, but this is not a linear proportion. Lenses of the same index can have somewhat different Abbe value. Standard plastic lenses have an abbe value of 58. Most high index materials have a much lower Abbe value. However, the effect of dispersion can be minimized by correct cent ration and by reducing the vertex distance, putting the edges of the lens farther from the normal line of sight.

Reflectance

Reflectance is the phenomenon of light reflection occurs at each of the lens surfaces. The result is the loss of lens transparency and undesirable reflections on the lens surfaces. The reflectance of the lens surface is calculated from the refractive index of the material. When the light is normal on the lens surface, the percentage of light reflected at each surface is given by:

$$\text{Reflectance} = 100 (n-1)^2 / (n+1)^2 \%$$

Therefore, a material of refractive index 1.5 has a reflectance of

$$100 (1.5 - 1)^2 / (1.5 + 1)^2$$
$$\text{Or, } 100 (0.5)^2 / (2.5)^2$$
$$\text{Or, } 100 \times (0.5 / 2.5)^2$$
$$\text{Or, } 3.9\% \text{ per surface.}$$

The higher the refractive index, the greater the proportion of light reflected from the surfaces. The unwanted reflection can be almost completely eliminated by applying an efficient anti-reflection coating, the need of which is more in higher index material.

Refractive index	% of light reflected
1.5	7.8%
1.6	10.4%
1.7	12.3%
1.8	15.7%
1.9	18.3%

Absorption

The amount of light which goes through a lens can be reduced because of absorption by the lens material. This is negligible in case of a non-tinted lens, but constitutes an intrinsic function of a tinted or photochromatic lens. Absorption of an ophthalmic lens generally refers to its internal absorption, i.e. to the percentage of light absorbed between the front and the rear lens surfaces. Lens absorption occurs according to Lambert's law and varies exponentially as a function of lens thickness.

Refractive Index

The refractive index of a transparent medium is the ratio between the velocities of the light in air to the velocity of light in the given medium and is denoted by 'n'.

$$n = \frac{\text{Velocity of light in air}}{\text{Velocity of light in the medium}}$$

This is a number, which has no unit and is always greater than 1. When the light passes from air to, say glass, i.e. rare medium to denser medium, the speed of their propagation slows down. How slowly they pass through the various transparent material is called the index of refraction of that material. Refractive index of material describes the ability to bend light. The higher the index of the material, the more it is able to bend light. A higher index of refraction results in a lower angle of refraction which means the bent light ray comes closer to the normal (perpendicular) line. In other words, for a given angle of incidence, the higher the index, the more light is bent. That is why "high index" lenses can be thinner for a given prescription compared to the lower index lenses although the reduction is not quite pro-rata **(Fig. 2.3)**.

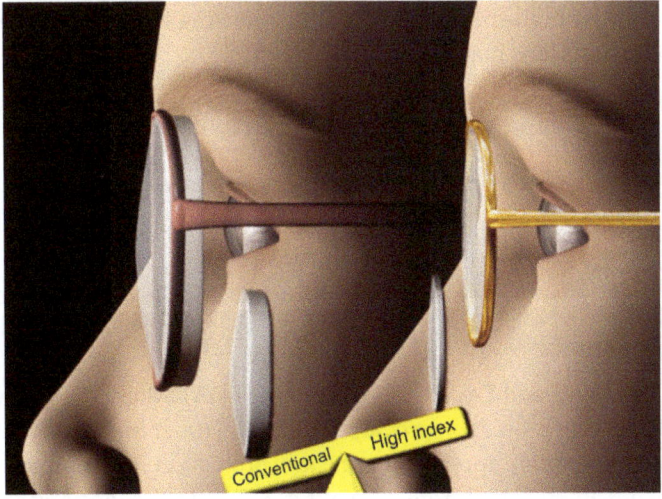

Fig. 2.3: Edge thickness reduces in high index concave lenses

As the velocity of light in a transparent medium varies with wavelength, the value of the refractive index is always expressed for a reference wavelength. In Europe and Japan, this reference is ne … 546.1 nm (mercury green line), whereas in other countries like USA it is nl … 587.6 nm (helium yellow line). The problem that this can cause is that a lens manufacturer may calculate the surfacing curves for a lens base on one refractive index, while the user may measure the same lens on a focimeter calibrated for another. But the difference only changes the 3rd decimal of the value of the index. So in fact it has no real effect.

An index over 1.74 can be described as "a very high index", 1.54 to 1.64 as "mid index" and anything lower is "normal index" if we assume that nothing less than 1.498 will be dispensed.

Mechanical Properties

Mechanical properties define values relative to mass, volume and dimension, and resistance to deformation and shock.

Specific Gravity

Specific gravity is the measurement of physical density or weight of the material in grams per cubic centimeter. In designing light weight lenses, a lens material with low specific gravity will produce a lighter lens. Reduction of weight improves wearing comfort, and eliminates the indentations from nose pads that are produced by wearing heavy glasses. However, low density does not always mean a lighter lens – the amount of material depends on the refractive index and the minimum thickness. But low specific gravity is very important for prescriptions that require high powered plus or minus lenses. Patients with high power prescriptions are usually advised to use higher index glasses. Although they offer thinner lenses, they are not necessarily more comfortable to wear because of their high specific gravity. The following table shows the specific gravity of various lens materials:

Material	Refractive index	Specific gravity
Polycarbonate	1.590	1.20 gram/cc
CR_{39}	1.498	1.32 gram/cc
Crown glass	1.523	2.54 gram/cc
High index glass	1.60	2.63 gram/cc

Impact Resistance

In 1971, the Food and Drug Administration (FDA) adopted a procedure to ensure the level of protection provided to the consumer for "street wear". More stringent standards are applied for industrial protection. The standard involves dropping a 5/8" steel ball from a height of 50" onto the lens and the lenses that survive this test are deemed impact resistant. The implementation of this standard in the USA led to increased use of hard resin lenses. Only a sample of hard resin lenses is needed to be tested for impact resistance, whereas every glass lens is needed to be tested. This accelerated the shift towards the plastic lenses **(Fig. 2.4)**.

Scratch Resistance

One of the straight features of glass lenses is abrasion resistance. Plastic lenses need to be coated with an additional resin to approach the scratch resistance of glasses. These resin coatings can be applied in a number of ways. Lenses may be dipped, or a thin layer of resin may be spun onto the lens surface. These coating layers are usually 5 micron thick.

While abrasion resistance is an important property for spectacle lenses, it is not crucial to the normal use of the product. Appropriate education of patients can assist them in avoiding situations where abrasion resistance becomes important, especially since the majority of scratches are put into the lenses by wearers themselves.

Initially plastic lenses were made from polymethylmethacrylate, which has poor abrasion resistance. A variety of other plastics and coated plastics have been used in the past 40 years, with scratch resistance steadily improving as the results of research and development are applied. These advances will continue and in near future, it is predicted that the abrasion resistance of plastic will get even closer to that of glass.

Thermal Properties

Thermal properties are those properties of ophthalmic lens material which is related to its conductivity to heat. In other words, these are the properties

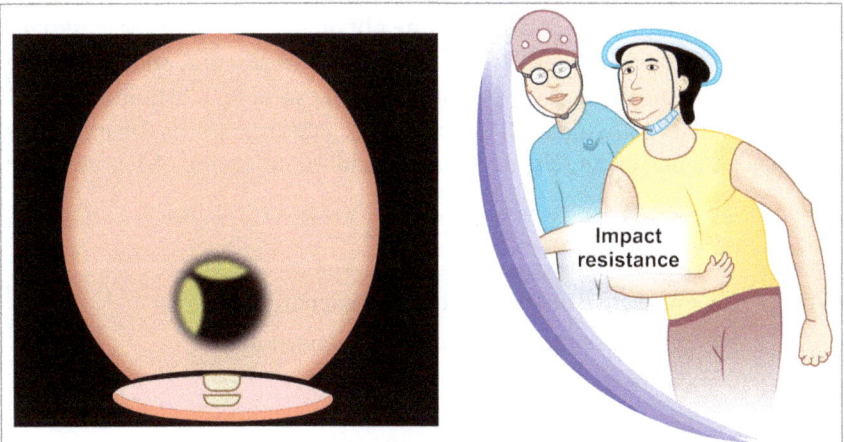

Fig. 2.4: Drop ball test for impact resistance

which are exhibited by a material when the heat is passed through it. Linear expansion coefficient is one of the important thermal properties of ophthalmic lens material. A moderately low expansion coefficient means that lenses can undergo, without any great risk of damage, treatments such as tempering and vacuum depositing of tinted or anti-reflection coatings, all of which expose them to high temperature cycles. Likewise, moldings have to be capable of resisting machining operations where they are exposed to considerable increase in temperature followed by sudden cooling.

Chemical Properties

Chemical properties of ophthalmic lens material refer to those properties that can be observed when they are being exposed to various acidic agents, alkaline agents and other organic solvents. International standards also require testing to determine fire resistance of materials used to manufacture lenses.

Electrical Properties

Electrical properties characterize effects of electromagnetic waves and electricity on the materials. They are governed by complex laws of physics.

Optical lenses modify the direction of the propagation of light and the relative spectral energy distribution of ultra-violet, visible and infra-red. Therefore, the above properties are the essence of optical lens material and need to be controlled very strictly. Optical lenses must be free from internal defects and strain, with a high standard of homogeneity. They must be produced within tight limits with respect to each property.

■ CURVE VARIATION FACTOR

Curve variation factor shows the variation in surface power when the lens material is other than crown glass. It is useful to know the likely change in the volume and thickness which will be obtained when another material is compared with the standard crown glass. This information enables a direct comparison in the thickness to be obtained. For example, 1.70 index materials have a CVF of 0.75D, which will be about 25%, if this material is substituted for crown glass. For a given refractive and a standard index, the CVF is given by:

$$CVF = \frac{N_s - 1}{N_r - 1}$$

Where, N_s = refractive index of standard lens material.

N_r = refractive index of substituting lens material.

CVF in above example would be:

$$CVF = \frac{1.523 - 1}{1.70 - 1}$$

$$= \frac{0.523}{0.700}$$

$$= 0.747 \text{ D}$$

$$= 0.75 \text{ D approx.}$$

Alternatively, if we know the CVF, we can use the same to convert the power of the lens that is to be made into its crown glass equivalent. This is done simply by multiplying the power of the lens by the CVF for the material. For example, to make – 10.00D in 1.70 index lens, the crown glass equivalent would be 0.75 x – 10.00 D, i.e., – 7.50 D. In other words the use of 1.70 index material would result in a lens that has a power of – 10.00 D, but in all other respect looks like a – 7.50 D lens made in crown glass.

OPHTHALMIC LENS DESIGN

Lens Designing is the process of defining the lens forms. Lens form represents the shapes of two surfaces of a lens. The shapes of the two surfaces are given by their curves. The curves so designed may be either one single curve across the entire lens surface or multiple curves on one surface and the forms may be:
- Bi-convex
- Bi-concave
- Meniscus
- Plano-convex
- Plano-concave
- Aspheric
- Atoric
- Lenticular

Or, any other form of lens that improves its optical performance by minimizing the effect of lens aberrations. A complicated lens form may not be so specifically defined. It may be defined by mathematical equation.

There are two different approaches as shown in **Flowchart 2.1**, that can be adopted to design ophthalmic lenses:

Mathematical Process

This lens designing process for a lens involves calculation of off-axis errors in terms of sagittal and tangential errors from the lens for each principal meridian using computer software. A desired goal is set to achieve the optimum lens

Flowchart 2.1: Ophthalmic lens design approaches

| Mathematical process | Laboratory simulation |

design. Calculation of the sagittal and tangential errors of each principal meridian for different sets of front and back lens curves are mathematically analyzed as the surface curves are altered. Best combination is determined that provides the best off-axis optical quality.

Laboratory Simulation

Various combinations of lens forms are tried in front of simulated far point sphere of human eye. This far point sphere is the optical conjugate of the retina of the unaccommodated eye in rotation. The image of an object point formed on this sphere is usually a blurred spot instead of a sharp point due to aberrations of the lens. In order to measure the quality of the image of any object point, the lens designer sends a set of selected light rays that enter the simulated eye after refraction through the lens. The image quality is determined by the shape and size of the blur spot formed on this sphere. The lens designers strive to improve the quality of image by working upon the shape and size of image. To achieve the desired goal they manipulate the effect of various lens' optical aberrations in the best possible way. Best design is achieved when near perfect image quality is determined. Finally, an optimal choice is made to balance between optics and cosmesis.

The goal of ophthalmic lens design is to give the patient clear vision at all distances through any portion of the lens. The primary responsibility of the lens designer is to design a lens which provides maximum dynamic field of vision for the patient through all its portions. The lens designer has a very limited degree of freedom. Practical condition specifies lens materials, safety consideration fix lens thickness; fashion dictates lens position before the face, weight and cosmesis means only two lens surface can be used. In addition, various mechanical and optical factors impose further on the difficulties while designing the ophthalmic lenses.

The truth is that the central portion of the lens provides near perfect vision and is termed as 'On-Axis performance' of the lens. But the wearer has to look away from the optical center of the lens which results in wearer's line of sight makes an angle to the optical axis of the lens. It is only the peripheral or mid-peripheral portion of the lens that degrades and deforms the image quality and is termed as 'Off-Axis performance' of the lens. During off-axis viewing, the line of sight makes an angle to the optical axis up to 30 degree as the wearer observes the object in his visual field. All efforts of lens designing are directed towards improving the off-axis performance of the lenses.

The basic lens design is determined by the "base curve selection". The base curve of the lens is the curve that serves as the basis or starting point from where the remaining curves will be calculated. It affects the wearing comfort of the patient and also the cosmetic look of the lens. However, the concept of base curve is little confused in ophthalmic optics because of its innumerable definitions.

A dispenser defines the term "base curve" as the singular curve on the front side of the lens which he measures with the lens measure watch. He is most often guided by such measurement before beginning to work on the new prescription since this will dictate the curves that must be placed on the ocular surface to derive the proper prescription.

In case of semi-finished blanks the manufacturer is responsible for creating and finishing the front surface and from the front surface so created the laboratory calculates the variables needed to grind the back surface and thus creates the finished lens with the given prescription. The manufacturer designed curve on the front surface is defined as base curve.

In the earliest days, when the lenses were very simple, they were only ground as sphere. But with the advancement in the lens design, toric cylinder grinding was introduced. The type of lens produced was called cylinder lens, the two principal meridians of curvature were ground on the front side of the lens. The flatter of these two principle meridians of curvature was referred to as the base curvature of the toric surface **(Fig. 2.5)**.

Sometimes in early 1970s, the industry saw a dramatic change in the frame style. Consequently, bulgy front surface of the plus cylinder was found unsuitable. The hand edgers were pushing the 'V' bevel back and forth to achieve a good fit. The introduction of more automated system of edging commanded the industry to move the cylinder grinding to the back side. With minus cylinder grinding in place the single curve on the front of the lens became to be known as the base curve and the back side curves are known as ocular curves. This is now universally accepted definition of the base curve **(Fig. 2.6)**.

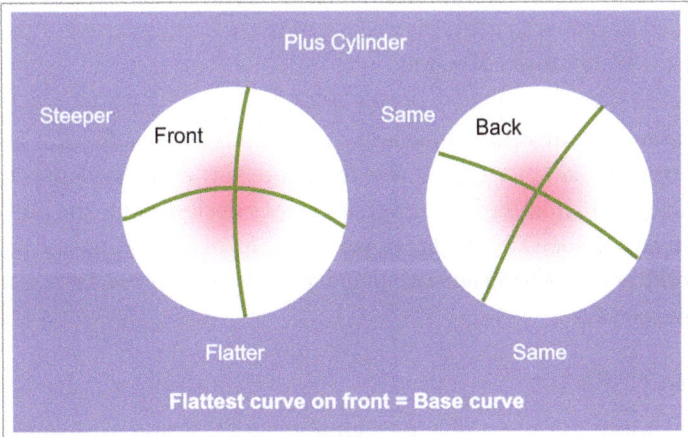

Fig. 2.5: Plus cylinder

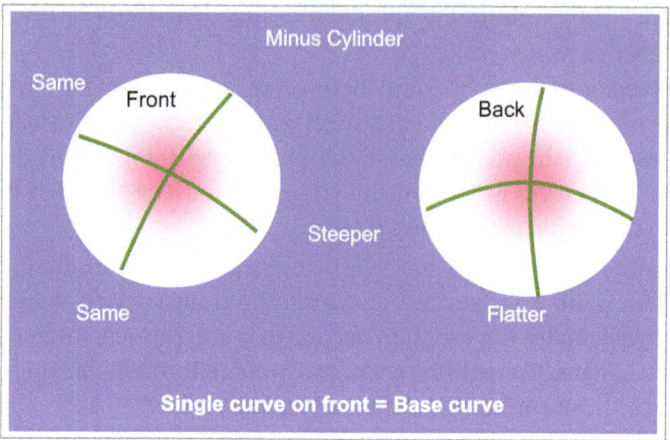

Fig. 2.6: Minus cylinder

The base curve of a lens may affect certain aspects of vision, such as distortion and magnification, and the wearer may notice perceptual difference between lenses with different base curves. Moreover, the wearer will adjust to these perceptual changes within a short span of time. That is the reason why some practitioners go with the idea of "match base curve" theory on the new prescription. However, patient with long eyelashes may be fitted with steeper base curves in order to prevent their eyelashes from rubbing against the back lens surface when their vertex distance is small. Also, some wearer with significant difference in prescription between right and left eyes may suffer from aniseikonia, or unequal retinal image size. Such case may require unusual base curve combinations in order to minimize the magnification disparity produced by the difference in the lens power.

Base curve is the starting point from where the remaining curves will be calculated. It serves as the basis to designate the lens form and it varies:
- For different ranges of power
- Also for the same range of power among different lens manufacturers.

Base curve of an ophthalmic lens can be altered to result in the best optics and cosmetic characteristics across the entire surface of the lens. Thus it is a basic design phenomenon for a spherical lens design. Since the power of the lens can be produced by infinite range of lens forms, choosing one base curve over another needs an extensive mental exercise on the two factors as shown in **Flowchart 2.2**.

Mechanical Factors

The maximum thickness of a lens, for a given prescription, also varies with the form of a lens in addition to lens material. Flatter lens forms are slightly

Flowchart 2.2: Factors affecting selection of base curve

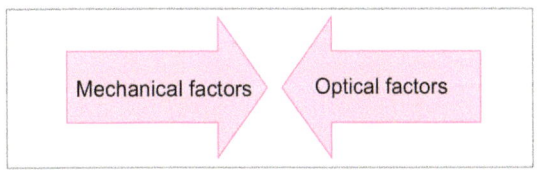

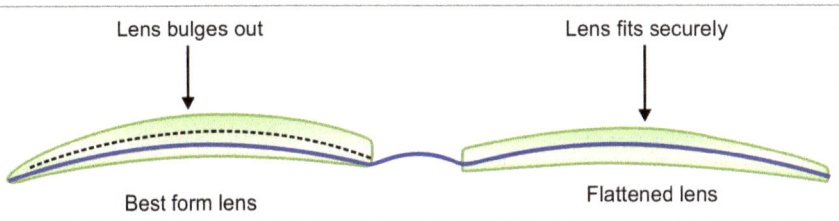

Fig. 2.7: Lens curvature

thinner than the steeper lens forms, and vice versa. Since the thinner lenses have less mass, they are lighter in weight as well. In addition to lens thickness, varying the lens forms will also produce significant difference in the sagittal depth or overall bulge. Plus lenses with flatter form do not fall out of the frame, which is very important with large or exotic frame shapes. Flatter lenses are cosmetically more appealing. Flatter lens in plus power is also associated with reduction in magnification and in minus power reduction in minification. This gives the wearer's eyes a more natural appearance through the lens **(Fig. 2.7)**.

Optical Factors

The mechanical factors for base curve selection clearly establish the advantage of the flatter lens. But the principal impetus behind the ophthalmic lens designing is their optical performance, not the cosmetic appearance. If the lens is designed flatter to make it look cosmetically appealing, it may perform optically poor. The whole idea behind choosing a correct base curve is to provide wider dynamic field of clear vision. Vision through the center of the lens may be relatively sharp, no matter whatever the lens form is, it is the vision through the periphery of the lens that will be greatly affected. However, the lens designed as the best form lens will not only look good, but will also minimize the disturbing lens aberration and will improve their off-axis performance, thereby ensuring the wider field of vision. If the lens looks good but performs poorly, it is bad lens. The patient's vision should always be held in highest regard. It is, therefore, important to balance optics with cosmesis while selecting the best form lens **(Fig. 2.8)**.

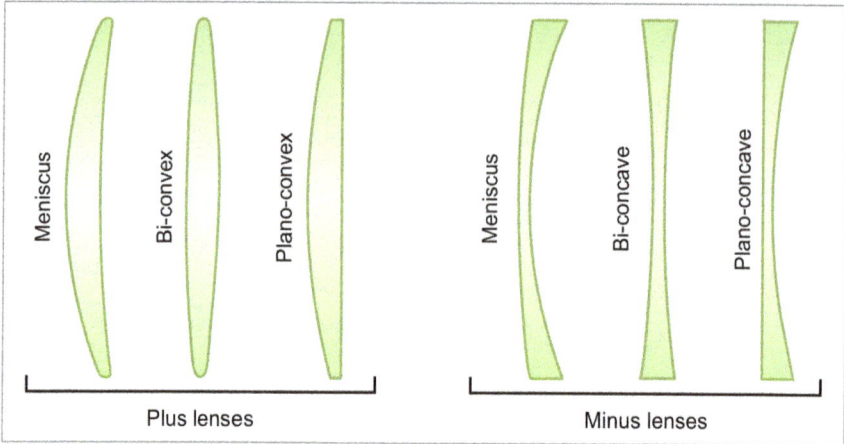

Fig. 2.8: Categories of lens form

The first step while selecting the correct base curve is to check the base curve of the existing glasses before manufacturing a new lens, if the patient is using any. Since the base curve will dictate the curves that must be placed on the ocular surface to derive the proper prescription, it is imperative to note the curves that the patient is currently wearing. If the patient is comfortable with the existing lenses and the new prescription is within a range of + or – 1.00D, then the base curve should generally be duplicated in the new pair of lenses. If the prescription is noticeably different, a slight adjustment in the base curve may be suggested **(Fig. 2.9)**.

While selecting a new base curve for a new wearer or adjusting the base curve of an existing wearer, it is important to understand how the selection of a curve will affect the finished product. Under ideal circumstances, a spectacle

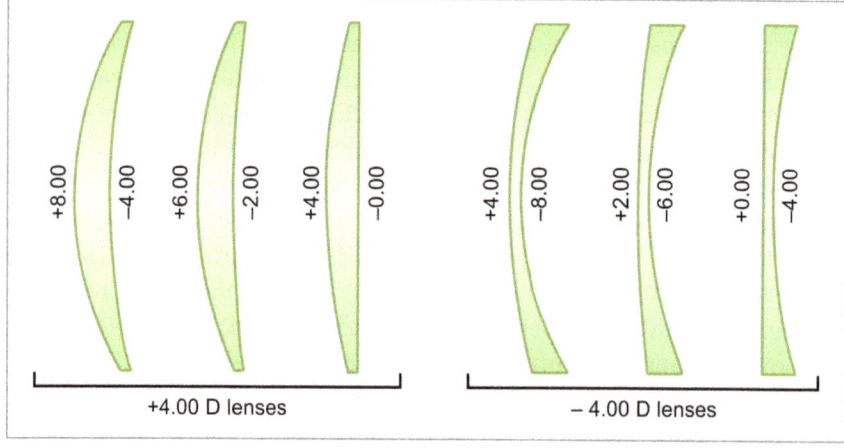

Fig.2.9: Lens form comparisons

lens would reproduce a perfect image on the retina. However, this is not always the case. The lens designer has to deal with varieties of aberrations which prevents perfect image through the lens. There are six types of aberrations that prevent perfect imaging through the spectacle lens.
1. Chromatic aberration
2. Spherical aberration
3. Coma
4. Oblique astigmatism
5. Curvature of field
6. Distortion

Chromatic aberration is caused because lens refracts the various wavelengths of light at different angles. Shorter wavelengths are refracted to a greater degree than longer wavelengths. The lens designer deals with this kind of aberration by selecting a lens material with low dispersive value. The small aperture of the pupil is effective in limiting the aberrant effect of comatic aberration and spherical aberration. Consequently, the lens designer pays little attention to these two types of aberrations. The effect of distortion does not alter the position of image, but merely affect its shape, to which brain adapts remarkably. The designers are left with oblique astigmatism and curvature of field. Oblique astigmatism is a real concern for the lens designers as it involves narrow beam of parallel rays that strike the lens at an oblique angle. Pupil does not limit the effect of oblique astigmatism. When a narrow beam of light rays strikes a lens obliquely, there is a tendency for the rays in the opposite meridians to focus at different points. The distance between the two points of focus equals the degree of astigmatism created. The presence of astigmatic error led the lens designer to work upon corrected curve theory. The idea was if the specific curvature can be controlled for specific correction, the effect of oblique astigmatism can be reduced. Such lenses are known as "Best Form Lens", and they are usually in meniscus form. The curvature of field refers to the phenomenon that the eye viewing an object through a lens does not create a true reproduction of the object. A flat plane may appear to look slightly curved. The effect is dependent upon the refractive index of the lens material and the curvature of the lens surfaces. In designing lens, the problem of oblique astigmatism and curvature of field are often closely related. However, field curvature is seldom totally eliminated.

The lens which is centered perfectly and also fits closer to the eyes and is able to keep the patient's vision within the central area of the lens reduces most of the troubles of these aberrations. Such a procedure may enable us to control some of the aberrations, but not all. Moreover, the lens designer does not try to concentrate on eliminating lens aberrations, but they intend to find a formulation that balances them out to reduce their effect. The science of creating the proper optical balance is referred to as "Corrected Curve Theory".

The corrected curve theory is the best form lens for a given prescription. Each lens designer has a slightly different application of the optical principles that control and balance the six lens aberrations. It is out of this optical reality that the theory of base curve selection has its application. Lot of mathematical computations are needed to determine the most suited base curve to the prescription. The computations are based on delivering the best optics in any given situation and not just creating the flattest profile. A flatter lens may look good, but the wearer may complain about compromised optics. Corrected curve theory outlines an effective method for minimizing the effect of lens aberrations. Only one combination of curves will yield the best form and will focus light to the clearest image by eliminating the most amounts of lens aberrations, and if the dispenser combines proper base curve along with good fitting and perfect optical center, the result is good cosmetics and great optics.

There are many corrected curve theories—the ellipse, a graphical representation developed by Marcus Tscherning shows the best base curve for every prescription to minimize the effect of oblique astigmatism **(Fig. 2.10)**. It says that there is a range of power from about -23.00 D to about +7.00 D that can be made free from particular aberration. Outside this range there is no perfect base curve. He demonstrated that there are two recommended best form base curves for each lens power. Tscherning's ellipse is the locus of points that plot out the recommended front curves for each lens power. The two curves are "Ostwalt bending" which is flatter form and "Wollaston bending" which is the steeper form. The flatter form is most commonly employed today. Wollaston is a deep curve form and is difficult to produce. For example – 5.00 D lens requires a back surface power in the region of -9.50 D in Ostwalt form, whereas the Wollaston form needs a back surface power in the region of -22.00 D, made with a lens of 1.523 refractive index.

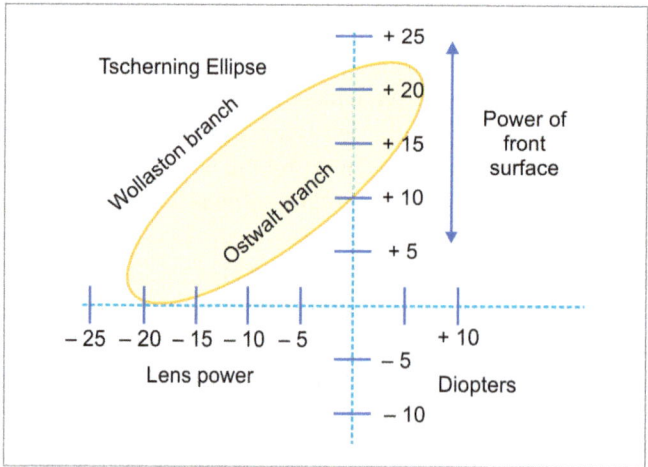

Fig. 2.10: Corrected curve theory

Table 2.1: Vogel's formula

Power	Base Curve
10.00	10
8.00	
6.00	8
4.00	
2.00	6
Plano	
-2.00	
-4.00	4
-6.00	
-8.00	2
-10.00	Plano

Another method for matching the best curve for a given lens comes in the form of Vogel's Formula as given in **Table 2.1**.

When selecting the proper base curve for a given prescription it is important to follow some rules. Keep basic prescriptions (+2.00D to -2.00D) on 6.00 dioptre base curve and adjust higher powers in plus to steeper front curves and while moving greater minus powers to flatter front curves.

The rule of thumb for selecting an appropriate base curve is take the spherical equivalent of the given prescription, if it is plus, add + 4.00 to that power to get a good approximate base curve. If it minus, add + 8.00 to that power to get a good approximate base curve.

Example

Given prescription + 4.00 Dsph + 1.00 Dcyl × 90
Spherical equivalent + 4.50 D
Base curve + 4.50 + (4.00) = + 8.50 D

Given prescription – 4.00 Dsph – 1.00 Dcyl × 90
Spherical equivalent – 4.50D
Base curve (– 4.50 D) + 8.00 = + 3.50 D.

This is the basis of spherical lens design. A lens so designed will yield good balance between vision and cosmetic look. However, the sagittal height of the lens will be more that will lead to more bulge and thicker appearance of the lens. Besides, off-axis performance will be significantly poor which will reduce field of clear vision through the lens. The designer got the solution in the form of aspheric lens design. Aspheric surfaces vary gradually in surface power from the center towards the edge, in a radial fashion. It means the asphericity is the same in every meridian of the lens. A spherical surface has the same curvature in any direction across the entire surface, whereas

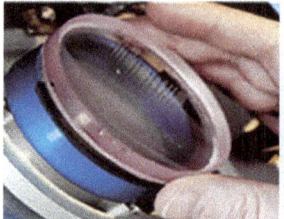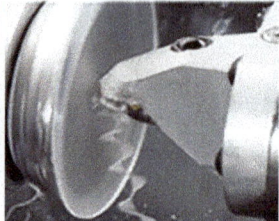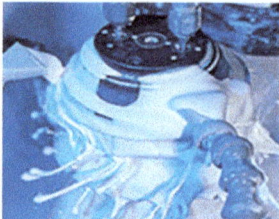

Fig. 2.11: Digital lens surfacing

aspheric surface becomes progressively flatter or, steeper away from the center of the lens, i.e., the tangential meridian of the lens. Aspheric surface changes very little around the circumference of the lens, which is the sagittal plane of the lens perpendicular to the tangential plane. The difference in surface curvature produces surface astigmatism which neutralizes the oblique astigmatism produced by looking through the off- axis portion of the lens. Before the appropriate aspheric design is determined, the lens designer must first decide upon the base curve for the lens. Aspheric lenses generally use flatter front curves and then determine the asphericity required for the particular choice bending to eliminate oblique astigmatism. The lenses so made do not provide better vision than the best form lenses but they do provide equivalent vision. Nevertheless, asphericity gives lens designers the freedom to optimize just about any base curve for the chosen focal power or range of powers.

With the new Free-Form Lens Designing process in place the lens manufacturer uses digital technology to produce lenses **(Fig. 2.11)**. The process of lens surfacing starts using block of lens material. The block is cut using a single point cutter that removes material from the spinning blank to create a desired surface. The cutter is precisely controlled by motors which follows a path contained in the form of a digital file. The resulted finished surface can be virtually any shape or curve with the potential for great precision. The process enables lenses to be produced to 0.01 D power accuracy and can reduce lens aberrations and yield less peripheral distortion and peripheral blur.

No lens is perfect. A well design lens is the most perfect in that they achieve a best form that minimizes the effect of most lens aberrations. In this way it can be said that lens designing is the process in which an optimal choice is made from available options to provide the best possible form of lens.

Chapter 2: Ophthalmic Lens Material and Design

 Multiple Choice Questions (MCQs)

1. What is being mixed in the glass lens material to give rise to tints?
   a. Oxides
   b. Sulphur
   c. Potassium
   d. None

2. A lens made of glass material has an index of 1.70 without an anti-reflective coating. If the lens is clear, what is the percentage of light transmission entering the patient's eyes if 100 percent of light is incident at the front lens surface?
   a. 84 percent
   b. 87 percent
   c. 90 percent
   d. 93 percent

3. What does the Abbe Number of an ophthalmic lens material denotes?
   a. Represents the relative degree of distortions generated while looking through the off-center areas of lens
   b. Represents the physical properties of the lens material to show the degree of hardness
   c. Represents the light transmissibility factor through the lens material
   d. Represents the weight of the lens material

4. Which of the following properties denotes that the lens material is relatively heavier?
   a. Refractive index
   b. Specific gravity
   c. Abbe number
   d. None of the above

5. Which of the following is true about CVF?
   a. CVF shows the variation in surface power when the lens material is other than standard crown glass
   b. CVF shows the variations in focal power of lens when the lens material is other than standard crown glass
   c. CVF shows the variations in vergence power of lens when the lens material is other than standard crown glass
   d. None of the above

6. Abbe number of 60 is considered to have the least........................
   a. Spherical aberration
   b. Coma
   c. Chromatic aberration
   d. Oblique astigmatism

7. The lens form or lens profile of a spherical lens is predominantly determined by:
   a. Base curve selection
   b. Ocular curve selection
   c. Refractive index selection
   d. All of the above

8. What happens when the lens designer deviates from the rule of "best form lens" and produces flatter lens which provides thinner look?
   a. They induce unwanted aberration
   b. Blurred vision in the periphery
   c. Restricted field of clear vision
   d. All of the above

9. Why is the concept of "best form lens" so important?
   a. To provide clear vision from the center of the lens.
   b. To provide clear vision from the periphery of the lens
   c. To provide a wider field of clear vision
   d. All of the above

10. Which of the following is true about polycarbonate lens material?
    a. It is linear thermoplastic polymer with an amorphous structure
    b. It is more impact resistant and lighter than CR_{39}
    c. The material is very soft in nature and hence prone to scratches
    d. All of the above

Answers

| 1. a | 2. b | 3. a | 4. b | 5. a | 6. c | 7. a | 8. d | 9. c | 10. d |

Chapter 3

Spherical Lenses

Spherical lens is the lens whose surface has the shape of the surface of a sphere (**Fig. 3.1**). A sphere is a solid with all its points lying at the same distance from the center and the radius of curvature is same in the entire meridian from center to the periphery. When you cut the sphere from any portion, it gives a structure with two surfaces having two specific curvatures on its both sides.

The curvature of the spherical surface is dictated only by its radius of curvature which controls how steep or flat the surface would be. The larger the radius of curvature, the flatter is the curvature of the surface and shorter the radius of curvature, the steeper is the curvature of the surface. Thus, the curvature of a surface of spherical lens is inversely proportional to the radius of curvature and will increase in magnitude as the radius decreases in magnitude. This implies steeper curvature will produce stronger surface power (**Fig. 3.2**).

Spherical lens has similar power along its both the principal meridians, if we use the lens measure to find the curve on the front surface of a lens to be +6.00 D in both meridians and the curve on the back surface of the same lens to be -3.00 D in both meridians, we know the curves are spherical and determine the total power of the lens as depicted in **Figure 3.3**.

Parallel rays of light passing through the different areas of a spherical lens do not come to a focus to a common point, varying with the distance from the center of the lens. Peripheral rays bend more than the paraxial rays which create slight blurring of image.

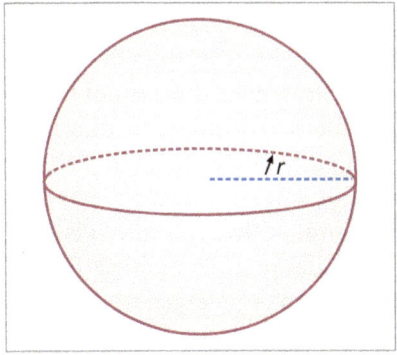

Fig. 3.1: Sphere

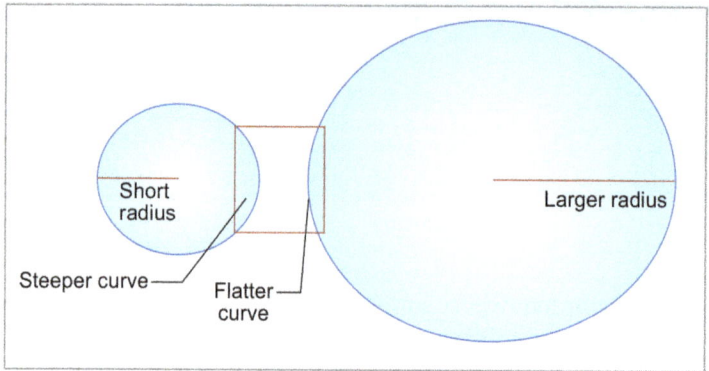

Fig. 3.2: Larger Radius results in flatter surface curve and Vice versa

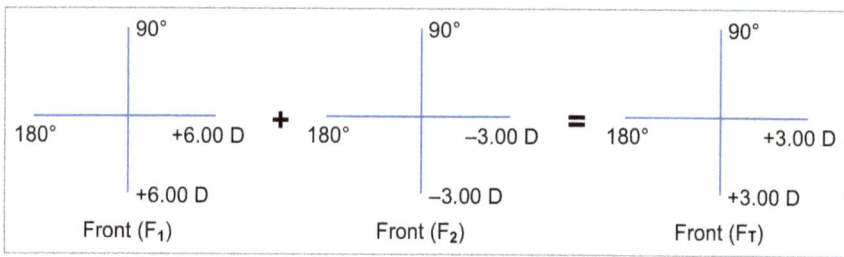

Fig. 3.3: Spherical lens power

There are various forms of spherical lens, some of them also have one plane surface. This is acceptable because a plane surface can be taken as part of a sphere with infinite radius **(Fig. 3.4)**.

Spherical surfaces are either convex or concave. A convex lens causes convergence of incident light, whereas a concave lens causes divergence of incident light **(Fig. 3.5)**.

The total vergence of a spherical lens depends on the vergence power of each surface and the thickness of the lens. Since, most of the lenses used in ophthalmology are thin lenses, thickness factor is ignored **(Fig. 3.6)**. Thus, the total power of a thin lens is the sum of the two surface powers. Refraction can be thought of as occurring at the principal plane of the lens. In **Figures 3.7A and B** principal plane of the lens is shown as AB. The point at which the principal plane and the principal axis intersect is called the principal point or nodal point, of the lens which is denoted by N. Rays of light passing through the nodal point is undeviated. Light rays parallel to the principal axis is converged to or diverged from the point F, the principal focus **(Fig. 3.8)**.

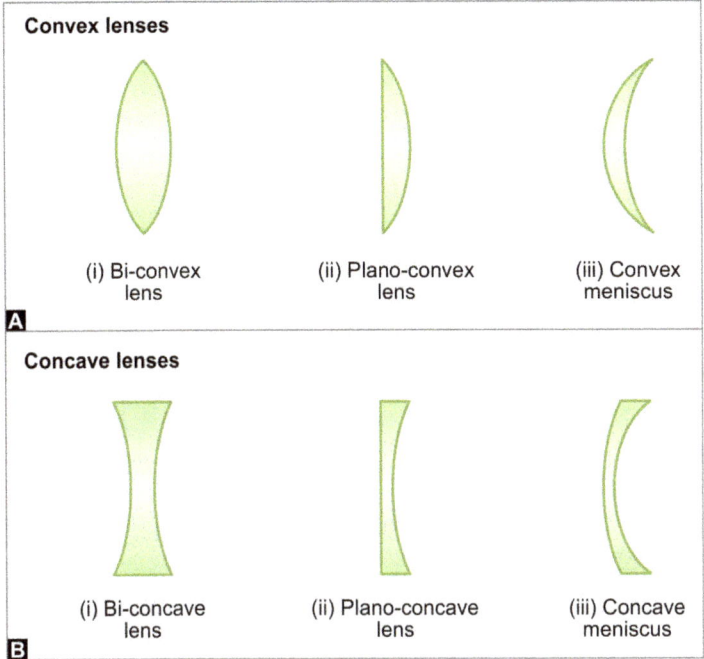

Figs. 3.4A and B: Basic forms of spherical lens

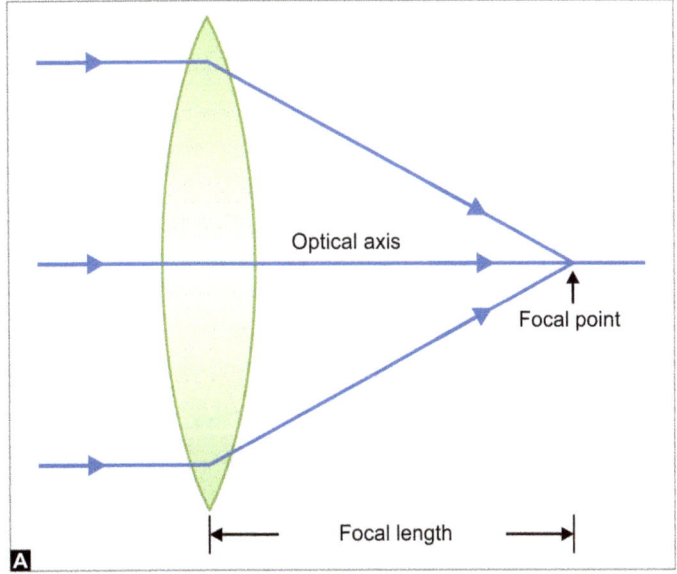

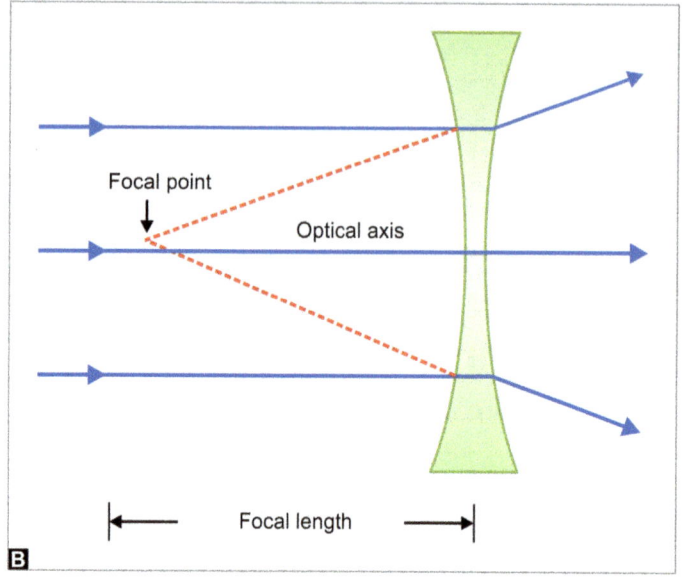

Figs 3.5A and B: Light passing through a lens obeys Snell's law at each surface: (A) Convex lens; (B) Concave lens

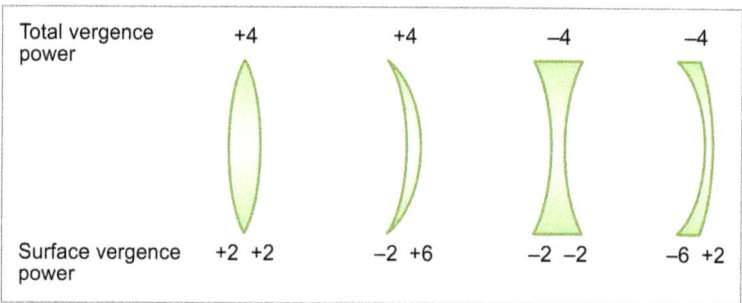

Fig. 3.6: Vergence power of thin lens

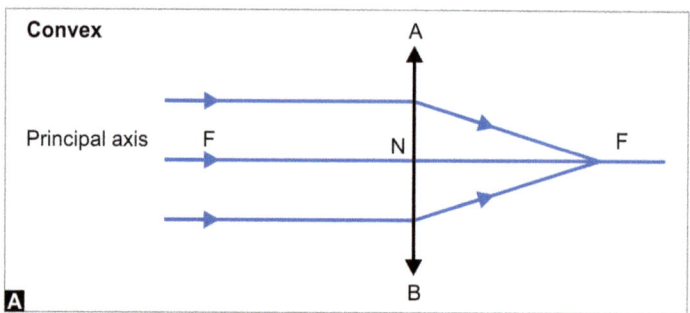

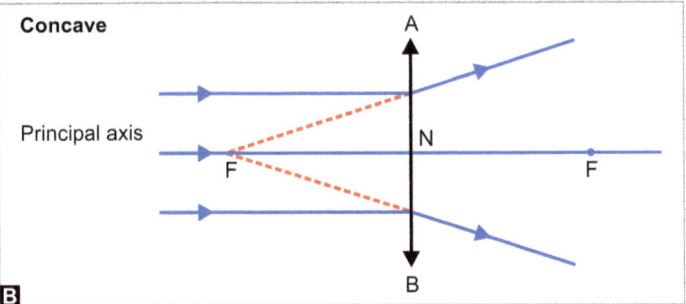

Figs 3.7A and B: Cardinal points of thin spherical lenses: (A) Convex; (B) Concave

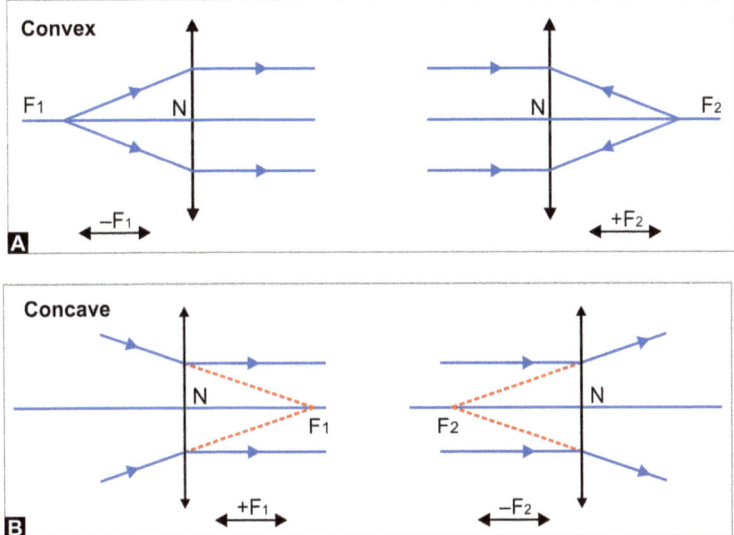

Figs 3.8A and B: The principal foci of thin spherical lenses

Since, the medium on both sides of the lens is the same, i.e., air, parallel rays incident on the lens from the opposite direction, i.e., from the right in Figure 3.7 will be refracted in an identical way. There is, therefore, a principal focus on each side of the lens, equidistant from the nodal point. The first principal focus F_1, is the point of origin of rays which, after refraction by the lens, are parallel to the principal axis. The distance F_2N is the first focal length. Incident rays parallel to the principal axis is converged to or diverged from the second principal focus - F_2. The distance F_2N is the second focal length. By the sign convention, F_2 has a positive sign for convex lens and negative sign for the concave lens. Lenses are designed by their second focal length. Thus, the convex or converging lenses are also called "Plus Lenses" and are marked with "+", while concave or diverging lenses are also called "Minus Lenses" and are marked with "–". If the medium on either side of the lens is the same, i.e. air,

DIOPTRIC POWER OF LENSES, VERGENCE

Lenses of shorter focal length are more powerful than lenses of longer focal length. Therefore, the unit of lens power, the diopter, is based on the reciprocal of the second focal length expressed in metres, gives the vergence power of the lens in diopters (D).

Thus, $F = 1/f_2$

Where F = Vergence power of lens in dioptres.

f_2 = Second focal length in metres.

So, in the above **Figure 3.9A** vergence at the lens is:

F = 1 / 0.25 = 4.00 D.

And in **Figure 3.9B** vergence at the lens is:

F = 1/ 0.10 = 10.00 D.

A converging lens of second focal length + 5 cm has a power of + 1/ 0.05 or + 20.00D, and a diverging lens of second focal length 25 cm has a power of – 1/ 0.25 or – 4.00 D.

SPHERICAL LENS DECENTRATION AND PRISM POWER

Rays of light incident upon a lens outside its axial zone are deviated towards (Convex lens) or away from (Concave lens) the axis. Thus, the periphery portion of the lens acts as a prism. The refracting angle between the lens surfaces grows larger as the edge of the lens is approached **(Fig. 3.10)**. Thus, the prismatic effect increases towards the periphery of the lens. Use of paraxial portion of a lens to gain a prismatic effect is called decent ration of the lens. Lens decent ration is frequently employed in spectacles where a prism is to be incorporated. On the other hand, poor centration of spectacle lenses, may produce an unwanted prismatic effect. The prismatic power of the lens is given by the formula:

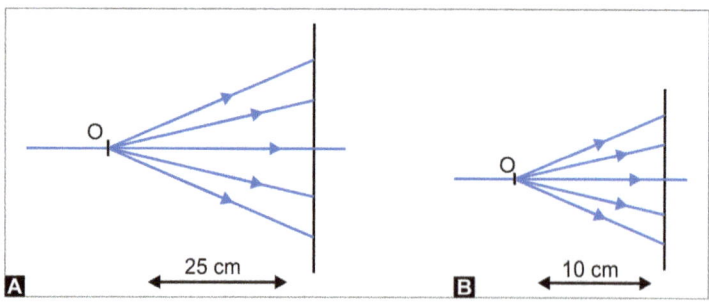

Figs 3.9A and B: Vergence of rays

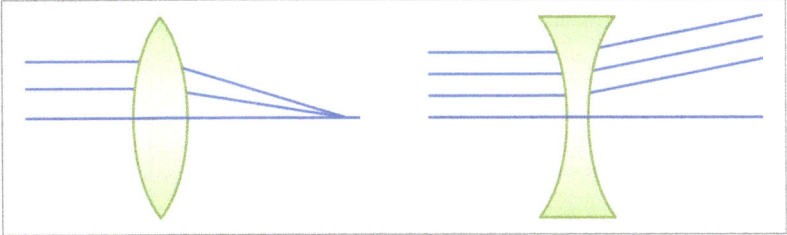

Fig. 3.10: Prismatic deviation by spherical lenses

$$P = D/d$$

Where, P = Prismatic power in prism dioptre.
D = Deviations produced by lens in cms.
d = Distance in metres.

The increasing prismatic power of the more peripheral parts of a spherical lens is the underlying cause of spherical aberrations.

DETECTION OF SPHERICAL LENS

It is possible to determine the spherical lens by studying the image formed when two lines crossed at 90º, are viewed through the lens. Spherical lens causes no distortion of the cross. However, when the lens is moved from side to side and up and down along the axis of the cross, the cross also appears to move. In the case of a convex lens, the cross appears to move in the opposite direction to the lens, termed as "against movement", while a movement in the same direction termed as "with movement" is observed if the lens is concave **(Figs. 3.11A and B)**. Rotation of a spherical lens has no effect upon the image of the crossed lines. The power of a lens can also be found using the neutralization method. Once the nature of the unknown lens is so determined, lenses of opposite type and known power are superimposed upon the unknown lens until a combination is found which gives no movement of the image of the cross line when the test is performed. At this point the two lenses are said to "neutralize" each other and the dioptric power of the unknown lens must equal that of the trial lens of opposite sign, e.g, a + 2.00 D lens neutralizes a – 2.00 D lens. To measure this accurately, the neutralizing lens must be placed in contact with the back surface of the spectacle lens. However, with highly curved lenses, this is not possible and an air space intervenes. It is, therefore, better to place the neutralizing lens against the front surface of the spectacle lens. Neutralization is, thus, somewhat inaccurate for curved lenses of more than about 2.00 D. An error of up to 0.50 D may be possible with powerful lenses. Nevertheless for relatively low power lenses, neutralization is still a very useful technique.

The Geneva lens measure can be used to find the surface powers of a lens by measuring the surface curvature **(Fig. 3.12)**. The total power of a thin lens

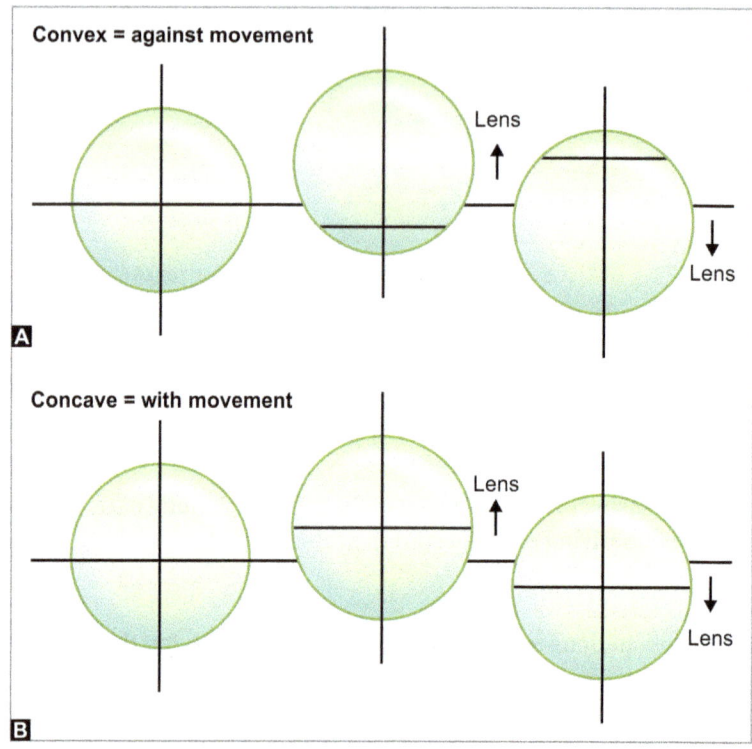

Figs. 3.11A and B: Movement test for detection of spherical lens

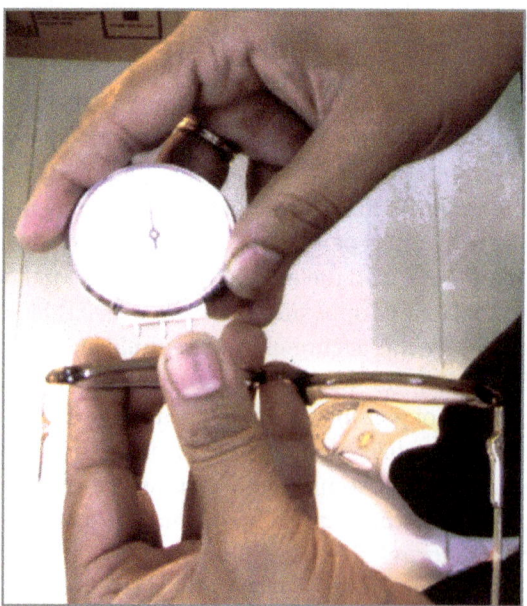

Fig. 3.12: Geneva lens measure watch

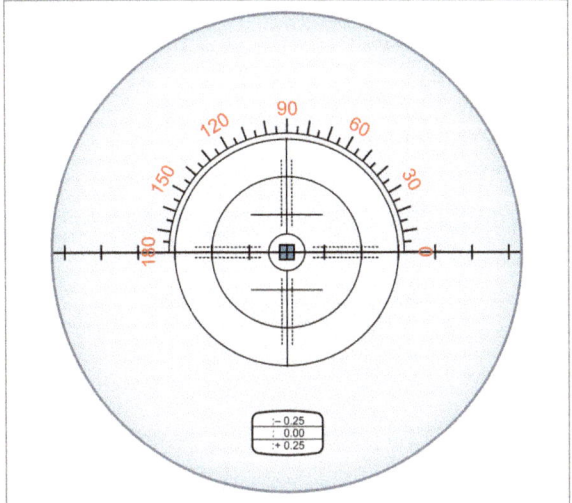

Fig. 3.13: Target as seen in Focimeter

equals the sum of its surface powers. However, the instrument is calibrated for lenses made of crown glass and a correction factor must be applied in the case of lenses made of materials of different refractive indices.

Focimeter is used to measure the vertex power of the lens. The image of the target is seen as a ring of dots when a spherical lens is tested **(Fig. 3.13)**.

Multiple Choice Questions (MCQs)

1. Which of the following is true about spherical lens?
    a. Both the principal meridians of the lens will have similar power
    b. Both the principal meridians of the lens will have different power
    c. One principal meridian will be stronger than the other in terms of lens power
    d. None of the above

2. Which of the following is true of about spherical lens?
    a. When a cross is viewed through the lens, there is no distortion of cross
    b. When the lens moves side to side, cross also appears to move
    c. When the lens is rotated, there is no effect on the image of the cross lines
    d. All of the above

3. Which of the following type of movement is observed when a convex spherical lens is moved against a cross target?
    a. Against movement
    b. With movement
    c. Rotational movement
    d. All of the above.

4. Which of the following type of movement is observed when a concave spherical lens is moved against a cross target?
   a. Against movement
   b. With movement
   c. Rotational movement
   d. All of the above.

Answers

| 1. a | 2. d | 3. a | 4. b |

Chapter 4

Astigmatic Lenses

In an astigmatic lens, all the meridians do not have the same curvature and a point image of a point object cannot be formed. The lens effectively gives a minimum power in one direction, gradually changing to a maximum power in the other, at right angle to the first. These meridians of minimum and maximum power are referred to as the principal meridians of the lens. There are two types of astigmatic lenses, namely cylinder lens and toric lens.

■ CYLINDER LENSES

Cylinder lens in most basic form is the sub-section of cylinder glass used to focus light in one dimension as opposed to spherical lenses which is used to focus light in two dimensions. They differ from spherical lenses in their geometrical shapes because of which additional specifications are needed to consider to express cylinder lenses as power meridian and axis meridian. Spherical lens has the same refractive power in all its meridians, whereas cylinder lens has maximum dioptre power in its power meridian and there is no power in its axis meridian which is perpendicular to the power meridian. A cylinder lens, therefore, is plane along its axis meridian and the radius of curvature is infinity. Perpendicular to axis meridian is the power meridian with finite radius of curvature depending upon refractive power. **Figure 4.1** shows a cylinder lens. The cylinder is positioned so that its axis meridian is horizontal in **Figure 4.1A** and vertical in **Figure 4.1B**.

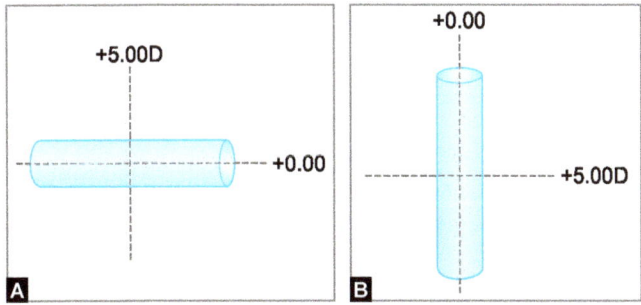

Figs. 4.1A and B: (A) Cylinder lens with no power along the horizontal meridian and +5.00 D along the vertical meridian; (B) Cylinder lens with no power along the vertical meridian and +5.00 D along the horizontal meridian

The image formation by cylinder lenses is not the same as spherical lenses. When the parallel rays of light from distant object point are incident upon convex plano cylinder lens, a line image will be formed, instead of point image, the image being elongated in the direction of power meridian as shown in **Figure 4.2**.

The behavior of a cylinder lens to light focusing depends upon orientation, i.e, how you place the axis meridian. If the cylinder lens is placed horizontally as shown in **Figure 4.1A**, the line image will be horizontal and if the cylinder lens is placed vertical as shown in **Figure 4.1B**, line image will be vertical.

A cylinder lens can be differentiated with spherical lenses as under:
- Both the meridians are curved in case of spherical lenses, whereas one meridian is curved and other is flat in case of a cylinder lenses.
- The point image is formed through a spherical lens, whereas a line image is formed through a cylinder lens.
- The orientation of cylinder lens determines its behavior to light, whereas orientation of lens does not affect its behavior to light in case of spherical lenses.

▮ NOTATION FOR CYLINDER LENSES AND ORIENTATION OF AXIS

A lens with purely cylinder power would be described as, say – 4.00 Dcyl (diopter cylindrical) in order to differentiate from the spherical one, which is described as – 4.00 Dsph (diopter spherical). As cylindrical surface is not rotationally symmetrical about the midpoint, a notation is required for their positioning in front of the eye. This is achieved by specifying the angle between the axis of symmetry of the cylinder and the horizontal. The universally used "standard" axis notation uses a protractor that reads anti-clockwise when looking at the face of the lens wearer. Angles upto 180 are used for the axis of cylinder, the full 360° protractor is only required for the base direction of prism. When describing a horizontal cylindrical axis, it is conventional to use the angle 180°, rather than zero. The orientation of cylindrical axis is opposite

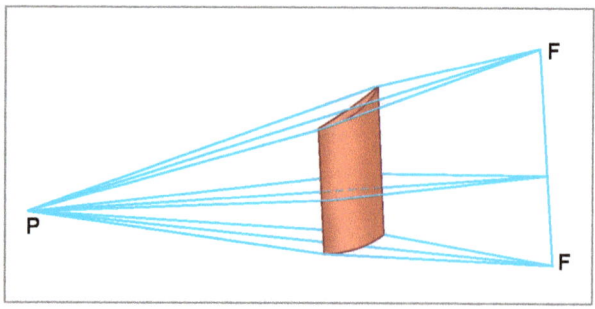

Fig. 4.2: The image of point object is not formed as point image, instead a line image is formed

the dispenser's side as compared with viewing the axis from the subject's side (**Figs. 4.3 to 4.5**).

A good way to recognize cylindrical axes from dispenser's side is to view the back of your left hand; the thumb will point to the 0° (**Fig. 4.6**).

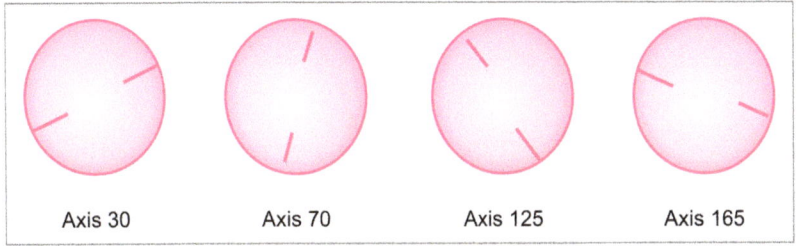

Fig. 4.3: Axis direction of astigmatic lens

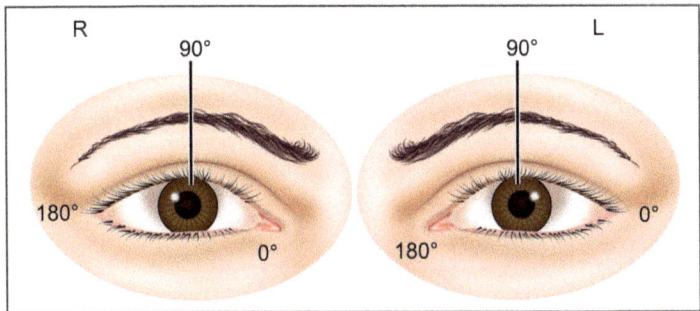

Fig. 4.4: Standard axis notation

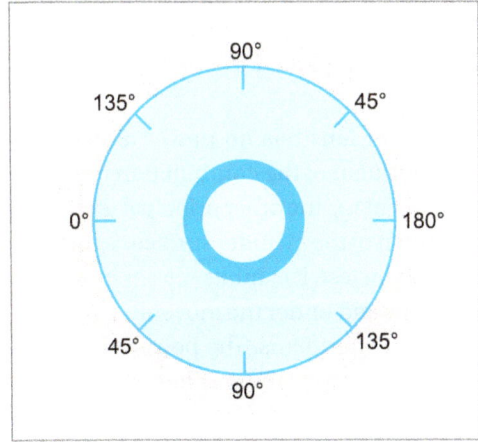

Fig. 4.5: Orientation of cylindrical axes on a protractor

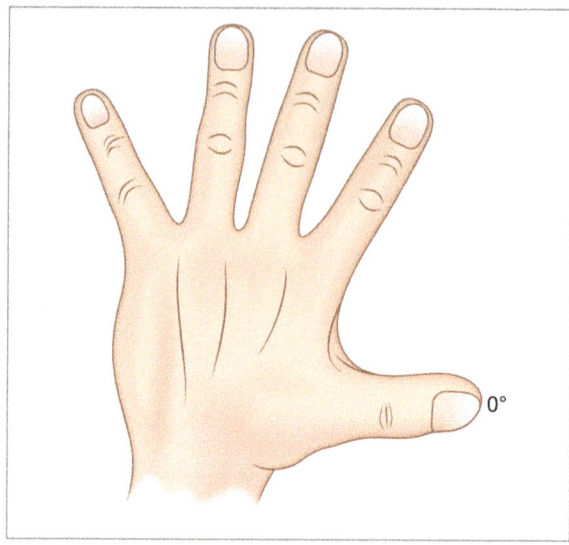

Fig. 4.6: Thumb will point to zero degrees

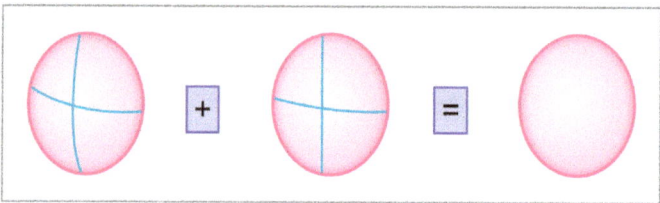

Fig. 4.7: Convex spherical surface combined with plano-convex cylindrical surface

TORIC LENSES

Toric lenses, also known as sphero-cylinder lenses can be explained as spherical lens that has been placed in contact with a plano-cylinder lens **(Fig. 4.7)**.

Since a plano-cylinder lens has no power along its axis meridian, the power along the axis meridian of the combination must result from spherical element alone. The power along the other principal meridian of the lens, at right angles to the axis meridian of the cylinder surface, is the sum of the sphere and cylinder. Under the rotation test, it exhibits scissor movement in the same way as a plano-cylindrical lens and under the movement test; it exhibits movement along each of its principal meridians. The power of a sphero-cylindrical lens is expressed by stating the power of the spherical component first, followed by the power of the cylindrical component, and finally the direction of the cylindrical axis. Thus, the specification:

$$-3.00 / -2.00 \times 90°$$

It signifies that spherical component of the lens is – 3.00D, the cylindrical component is – 2.00D and the axis of the cylindrical surface lies along the 90º meridian. On representing the power of the sphero-cylindrical lens by means of optical cross, the principal meridians show – 3.00D on vertical meridian and – 5.00D on the horizontal meridian as shown in **Figure 4.8**.

The pencil of light that results from refraction at an astigmatic lens is depicted in the **Figure 4.9**. Since the light does not focus as a point, the interval between two line foci is called the 'Interval of Sturm'. The best focusing occurs somewhere inside the interval of Sturm. This point is called the 'Circle of least confusion', and the complete envelop of the light near the circle of least confusion is called the 'Sturm's Conoid', named after the mathematician CF Sturm.

Figure 4.10 illustrates the toroidal surface of the sphero-cylinder lens. The lower power is usually referred to as the base curve of the surface and the higher power as the cross curve. In the plano-cylindrical surface, the base curve is along the axis meridian which is zero and the cross curve is simply the power

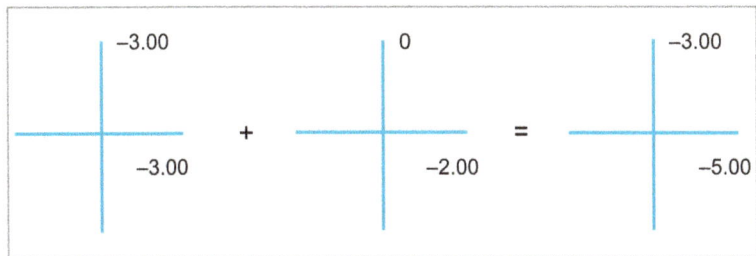

Fig. 4.8: Optical cross representation of – 3.00/– 2.00 × 90°

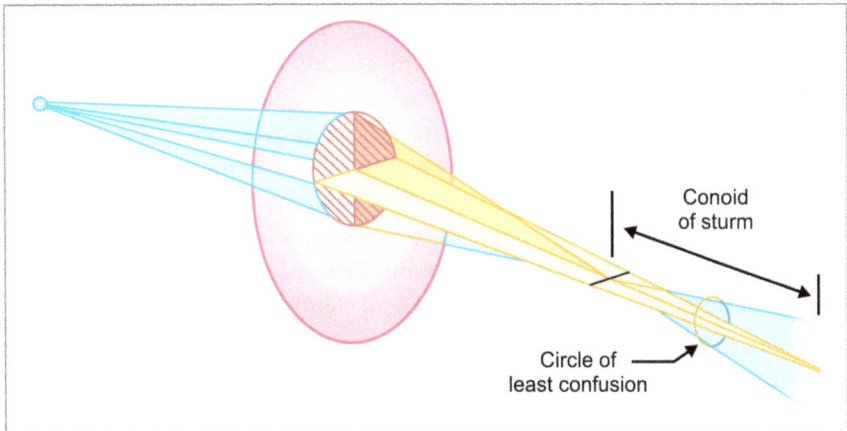

Fig. 4.9: Pencil of light results from retraction at an astigmatic lens

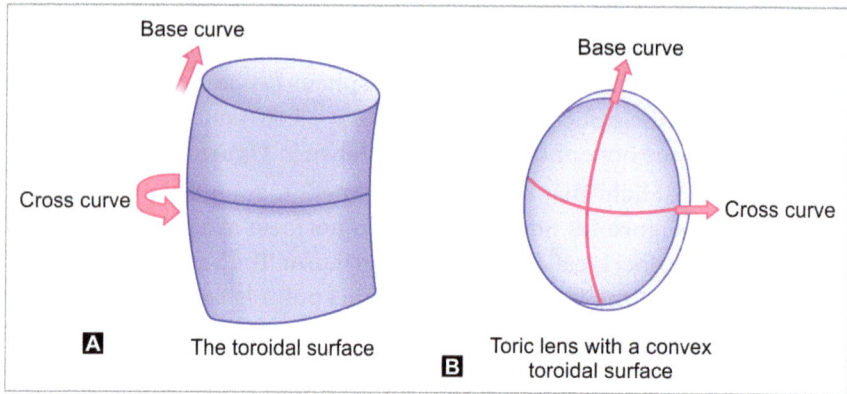

Figs. 4.10A and B: Toroidal surface of the sphero-cylinder lens

of the cylindrical surface. In case of the toroidal surface, the "axis meridian" is curved and the cylindrical power of the surface is the difference between the cross curve and the base curve.

■ DETECTION OF CYLINDRICAL LENS

Cylinder lenses are often referred to as cylinder or toric lens because of their out of round surfaces. In order to determine the cylinder lens and to detect its dioptric strength, hold the lens a few inches away from your eyes; sight a straight lined object, such as window or the door frame. Rotate the lens slowly as you would turn a steering wheel – first to the right (clockwise), then to the left (anti-clockwise). If a section of the door frame appears slanted as shown in **Figure 4.11** and **4.12**, it establishes that the lens under examination is a cylindrical lens. This is called "scissors like movement".

Next step is to find out two principal meridians of the lens. To do so continue rotating the lens and at one position on rotation, the frame of the door would not look slanted. This is one of the principle meridians. The meridian opposite to this is the other principal meridian. They are at 90 degree to each other. Now, neutralize both the meridians separately. If the movement in one meridian is nil, it is a plano-cylindrical lens and nil movement meridian is taken as the axis of the lens. Contrarily, if both the meridians show movement, it is a sphero-cylindrical lens. The weaker movement meridian is taken as the axis of the lens under observation. Now, neutralize both the meridians as before to determine exact spherical and cylindrical elements.

When a Cylinder lens is rotated against a crossline chart, the crossline also appears to rotate as shown in **Figure 4.13**.

Lensometer can also be used to determine the lens power of an astigmatic lens. The procedure is as under:

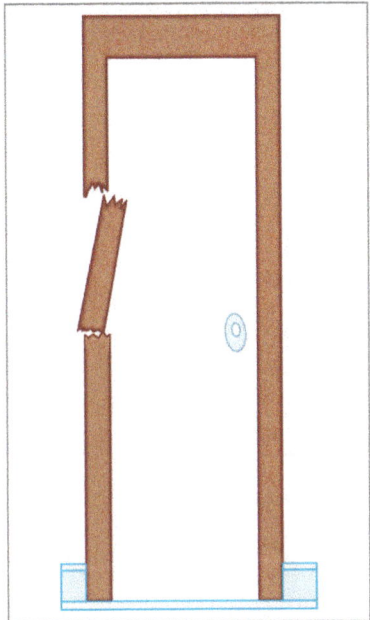

Fig. 4.11: Looking through a plano-cylinder, a section of the door's frame appears to be slanted

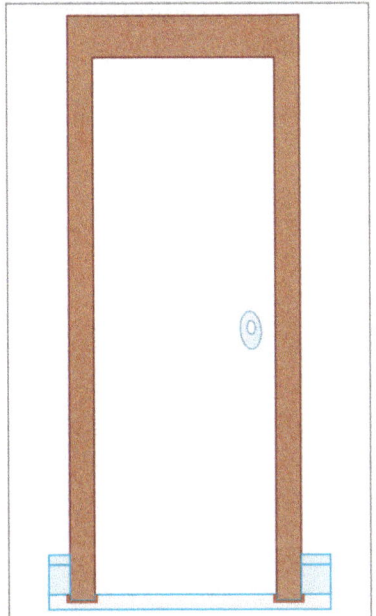

Fig. 4.12: Upon rotating the lens, a position will be found in which the door frame appears straight

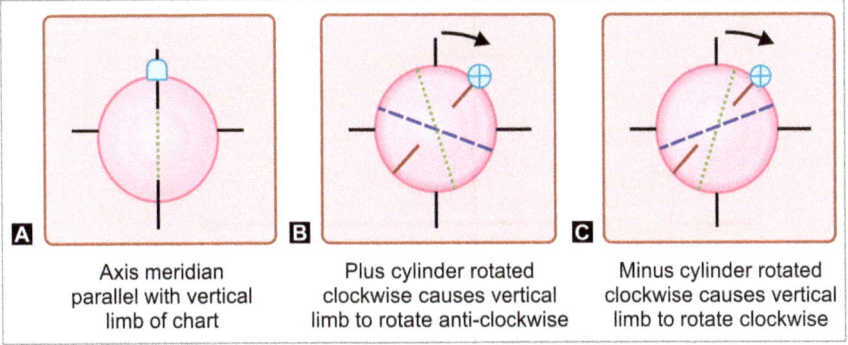

A	B	C
Axis meridian parallel with vertical limb of chart	Plus cylinder rotated clockwise causes vertical limb to rotate anti-clockwise	Minus cylinder rotated clockwise causes vertical limb to rotate clockwise

Figs. 4.13A to C: Rotation test to detect cylinder axis

- Place the lens on the lens stage and start from zero.
- Focus the target image by rotating the dioptre power knob.
- Read the dioptre power scale when the target image is cleared. This is taken as either plano for a plano-cylinder lens or spherical for a toric lens **(Fig. 4.14A)**.
- Now focus the target for other meridian by rotating the knob **(Fig. 4.14B)**.

- The difference between the second absolute value and the first is taken as cylinder.
- Align the cross line with the second focused point by rotating the axis wheel. The angle of the indicator shows the axis.

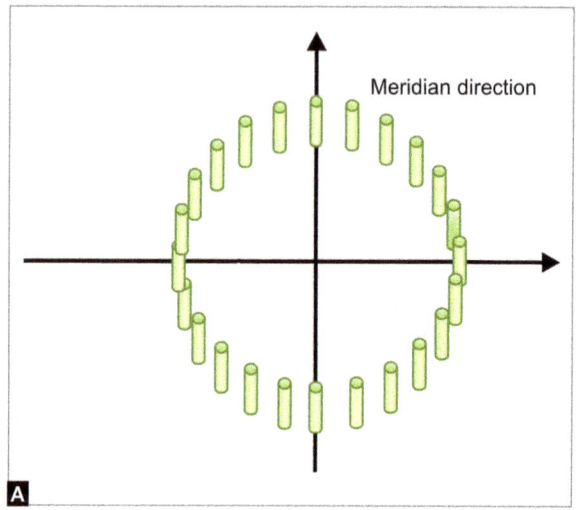

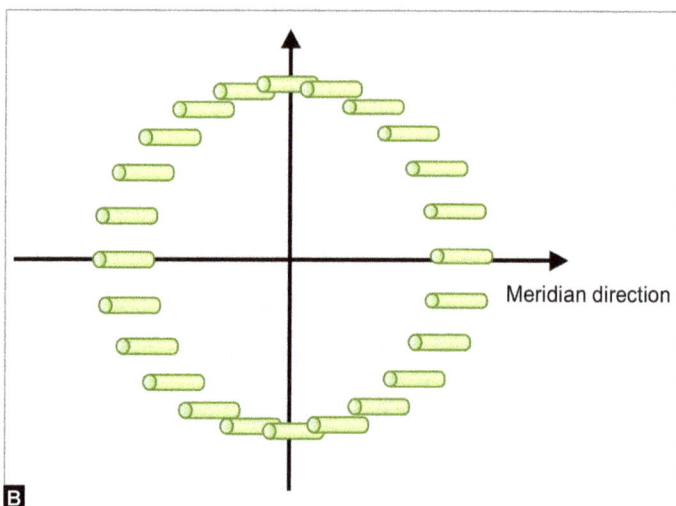

Figs. 4.14A and B: Circular star burst ring made of dots is seen as elongated lines in lensometer through cylinder lenses

Multiple Choice Questions (MCQs)

1. Which of the following is true about cylindrical power of the lens?
    a. Both the principal meridians will have same power
    b. Both the principal meridians will have different power
    c. The lens power will have vertical axis
    d. All of the above

2. Which of the following is true about plano-cylindrical lens?
    a. One meridian will have zero value and other will have some value
    b. Both the meridians will have same meridional values
    c. Both the meridians will have different meridional values.
    d. None of the above

3. Which of the following is true about sphero-cylindrical lens?
    a. One meridian will have zero value and other will have some value
    b. Both the meridians will have same meridional values
    c. Both the meridians will have different meridional values
    d. None of the above

4. Scissor like movement is seen in which type of lens?
    a. Spherical lens
    b. Cylinder lens
    c. Prism
    d. All of the above

Answers

| 1. b | 2. a | 3. c | 4. b |

Chapter 5

Prisms

When the rays of light pass through a piece of material as shown in **Figure 5.1**, travelling from air, it bends towards the normal. Then it leaves the material travelling back into the air and bends away from the normal. In this figure the sides of the material are parallel to each other, so the rays emerges travelling in the same direction as its original travel—it has been displaced, but not deviated.

In the **Figure 5.2**, the sides of the material are not parallel to each other, so the ray emerges travelling in a different direction than its original travel. This

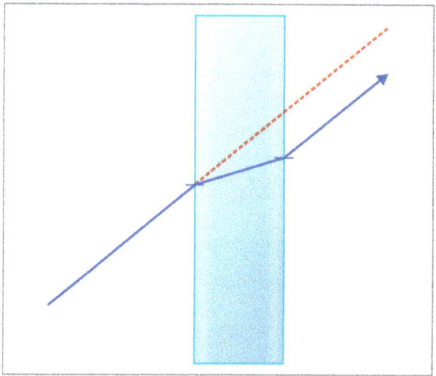

Fig. 5.1: The ray appears to be displaced

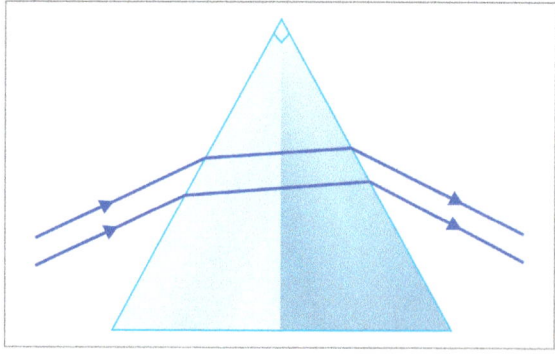

Fig. 5.2: Rays emerging, traveling in different direction

happens to every ray that passes through a refracting medium bordered by two plane surfaces which are inclined at a finite angle. The medium is called Prism and the angle between the two surfaces is called the apical angle or refracting angle. A line bisecting the angle is called the axis of the prism and the opposite surface is called the base of the prism.

The prism, therefore, can be defined as a piece of wedge-shaped transparent material whose refracting surfaces are not parallel to each other; instead they are inclined at a definite angle. The point at which the two surfaces meet is called apex and the surface opposite to apex is called base of the prism. All spectacle lenses have the effect of prism when viewed through a point away from the optical center. The further the away from the optical center, the greater is the prismatic effect.

A prism changes the direction of light without changing its vergence. However, the deviation of light causes the image to be relocated. Rays of light deviates towards base of the prism, whereas the image, when looked through the prism appeared to be displaced towards apex of the prism. The angle of deviation is called the prism power which is measured in prism diopter which denotes the amount of deviation produced by the prism. The power of prism may be expressed in terms of its apical angle which is denoted by prism degree. For a prism of 2 prism diopter gives a linear displacement of 2 cm at a distance of 1 meter, whereas prism of 2 prism degree is the measure of the apical angle produced at the apex of the prism. The deviations produced by prism depend upon its apical angle and the refractive index. For a crown glass having a refractive index of 1.523 a relationship can be drawn between prism diopter and prism degree saying that 1 prism degree can be considered equal to 1.75 prism diopter.

Look at the **Figure 5.3**, that shows a plano lens with prism. The base of the prism is thicker than any other portion and the plane opposite to base is the

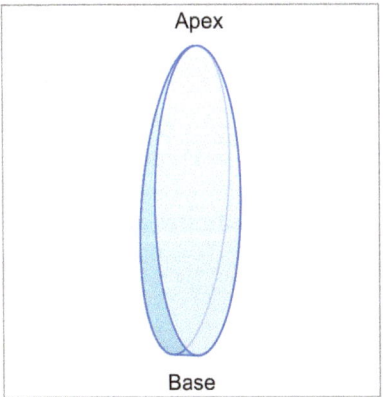

Fig. 5.3: Prism as it looks in an uncut lens

thinnest— known as apex of the prism. The thickest edge is exactly opposite the thinnest edge (provided prism has no power).

When the prisms are prescribed, the orientation of it, is indicated by the position of base, i.e., 'base - in', 'base - out' and so on. Light rays entering and leaving a prism are bent towards the base of the prism. This causes objects to be displaced away from the base of the prism towards its apex. Thus, if an object is viewed through a base down prism, it will be seen to be displaced upward. Similarly, objects appear to shift downward when viewed through a base up prism, to the right or left when seen through a base-out or base-in prism.

The amount by which a ray will be deviated when it passes through the prism depends on:
- The apical angle
- The index of refraction of the material
- The wavelength of the light
- The angle from which the ray approaches the prism.

CHARACTERISTICS OF PRISM

- A prism has a thickest edge, the base and a thinnest edge, the apex.
- A prism displaces the incident rays towards the base of the prism.
- A prism displaces the image towards the apex of the prism.
- A prism does not change the vergence of the rays.
- A prism does not magnify or minify the image.
- A prism also disperses incident pencil rays into its component colours.

DEVIATION PRODUCED BY PRISM

The deviation produced by a prism is measured in terms of prism dioptre and is given by the symbol Δ. A prism with a power of 1 prism dioptre deviates light by 1 cm measured at a distance of 1 metre from the prism. Similarly, a prism of 2 prism dioptre produces a deviation of 2 cm measured at a distance of 1 metre from the prism. The deviation so produced can be measured by following equation:

$$\text{Prism diopter} = \frac{\text{Deviation in cms}}{\text{Distance in metres}}$$

Example: If the light is deviated 6 metres at a distance of 3 metres, then the prism diopter would be:

$$P = \frac{0.6}{3} \text{ cm}$$

or, $P = 0.2\Delta$

PRENTICE RULE

Prentice's rule gives the amount of induced prism in a lens. Induced prism is defined as the prismatic effect created when the patient's visual axis does not pass through the optical center of an ophthalmic lens. Patient usually experiences this effect when looking through portion of a spectacle lens other than its optical center.

The Prentice Rule:

$P = cF$

Where P = Prism (Δ)

F = Lens Power in dioptre

C = Distance from the Optical center in cm

Thus a +5.00 D lens decentred by 4 mm or 0.4 cm downwards will produce a prismatic effect of 2 Δ base down.

As the above equation shows, the amount of induced prism is directly proportional to lens power and the distance from the optical center, the precise placement of the optical center is increasingly more important as lens power increases. In order to calculate the amount of induced prism, we can ignore the plus/minus signs of the prescribed lens power. It only matters to determine the direction of the prism's base. When we decenter a plus lens in any direction we create prismatic effect with base in same direction and when we decenter a minus lens in any direction, we create a prismatic effect with base in opposite direction.

PRISM ORIENTATION

Prism can be oriented in front of the eye using notations base-in or base-out, base up or base down when the directions are horizontal and vertical as shown in **Figure 5.4.** All other base directions require 360° notations as shown in **Figure 5.5**. Example: RE 2Δ at 160°.

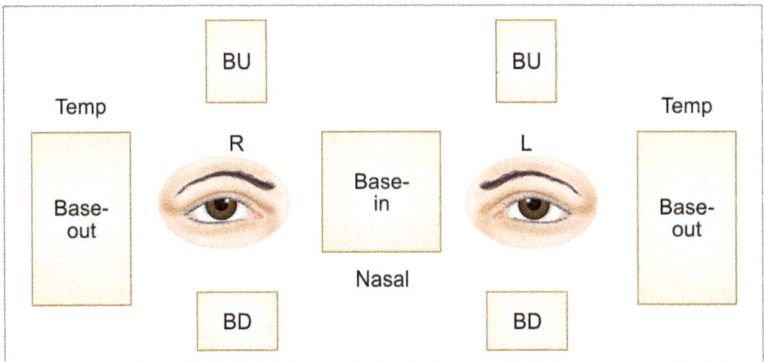

Fig. 5.4: Orientations of prism

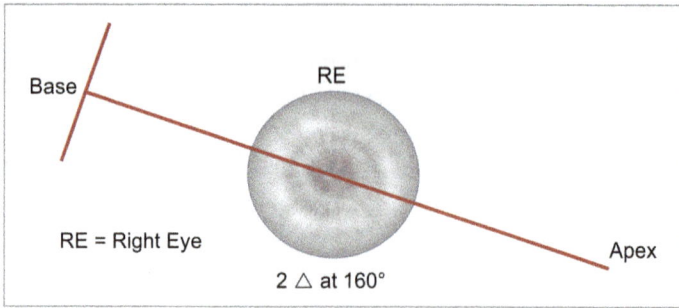

Fig. 5.5: Orientation of prism

BU = Base up
BD = Base down
Temp = Temporal
R = Right eye
L = Left eye

■ SPLITTING OR DIVIDING PRISM

When prism is prescribed, it is usually divided equally between the two eyes to:
- Distribute the weight more evenly.
- Reduce thickness of the intended lens.
- Minimize chromatic aberration.

For example, Right eye 3ΔIN causes right eye to deviate outwards by 3Δ. If we place 1.5ΔIN before each eye, the required total deviation will be still achieved. Therefore, RE 3ΔIN can be divided as RE 1.5ΔIN combined with LE 1.5ΔIN. Such a division in the horizontal meridian do not have to be equal in magnitude. For example:

Re Zero	LE 4 Δ OUT
R combined with L	
0.5Δ out	3.5Δ out
1Δ out	3Δ out
1.5Δ out	2.5Δ out
2Δ out	2Δ out
2.5Δ out	1.5Δ out
3Δ out	1Δ out
3.5Δ out	0.5Δ out
4Δ out	Zero

Exactly the same principle applies for BASE IN prism. While splitting the prism in vertical meridian, care must be taken to ensure correct base orientation. For example, RE 1.5Δ Up and LE 1.5Δ Down is not the same as RE 1.5Δ Down and LE 1.5Δ Up. The splitting can be done as under:

RE 3Δ UP	LE ZERO
R combined with L	
0.5Δ up	2.5Δ down
1Δ up	2Δ down
1.5Δ up	1.5Δ down
2Δ up	1Δ down
2.5Δ up	0.5Δ down
3Δ up	Zero

In practice usually splitting is done evenly.

TYPES OF PRISM

Prisms are used to change the path of the propagation of light. The following types of prisms may be used in practice:

Prism by Decentration

A larger uncut lens can be used to move the lens so that the optical center is no longer in front of the pupil and hence create a prismatic effect at the centre point **(Fig. 5.6)**. In case of anisometropia, the more powerful lens will need less decentration to create the same prismatic effect. Today a significant proportion of single vision lenses are aspherics where it is very difficult to decenter the lens to create prism at the center point. With the spherical curves, the effect away from the centre is a simple continuous curve, in case of an aspheric lens, the surface geometry is much more complex and the design has been calculated to work around the center of rotation of the eye. If an aspheric lens is decentred

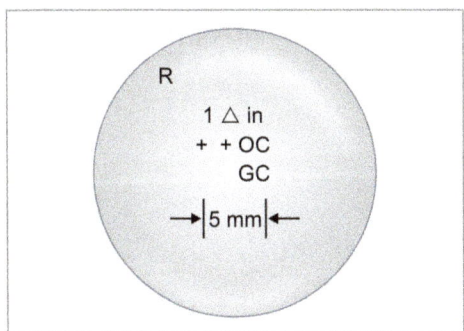

Fig. 5.6: Decentration in GC = Geometrical center, OC = Optical cen

then the vision would be compromised, especially in the periphery opposite to the direction of decent ration. On an aspheric lens, using prolate ellipsoid surface, the actual surface power reduces from the center to the edge, the outcome of this flattening is the reduction of prismatic effect in comparison with the same point on a spherical lens. The flattening is not the primary effect of aspheric lenses but is the side effect of the surface geometry.

Worked Prism for Decentration

Worked prisms work in exactly the same way, but creates the opposite effect. Here, we are looking to avoid creating unwanted prismatic effect at the center point. When the uncut is not available in the required diameter, working a prism on the lens will move the optical centre across the uncut lens creating a greater effective diameter **(Fig. 5.7)**.

Prescribed Prism

The prisms may be prescribed to create a desired effect upon the binocular balance of the eyes; this may be to reduce the visual stress to a tolerable level where a phoria is involved or to relieve a convergence insufficiency.

Differential Prism at Near

In case of anisometropic population looking away from the optical center create a loss of contrast and reduction in visual acuity which causes a breakdown in binocular vision and diplopia due to the induced differential prismatic effect. For a single vision spectacle wearer, this can be kept in check by looking through the optical center, but for the multifocal wearer, this differential prism must be tackled. In a multifocal lens, the zone that is used to read lies below the distance visual zone. The center of the near visual zone, is usually taken to lie somewhere around 8 mm below DVP and 2.5 mm inwards. Assuming that the impact of pantoscopic tilt has been taken care of, the prismatic effects generally differ at the visual points. The difference in the prismatic effects between the eyes is called differential prism and requires the eyes to rotate by different amounts to maintain binocular single vision of the object of regard. Remember eyes can cope with

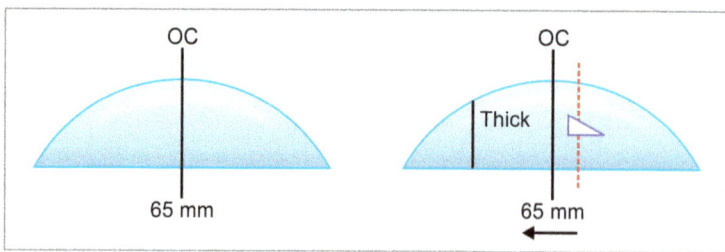

Fig. 5.7: Worked prism

quite big horizontal differential prismatic effects, but the great discomfort arises if the eyes encounter vertical prism, as it quickly produces diplopia. The eyes can cope with maximum 2∆ of vertical differential prismatic effect for longer hours.

Take for example a prescription in RE − 3.00Dsph and LE − 6.00Dsph, the vertical prismatic effects that the subject encounters at points 8 mm below the distance optical centres are RE 2.4∆ base down and LE 4.8∆ base down. The differential prismatic effect between the eyes is 2.4∆ base down in the left eye. This prevents comfortable binocular vision and hence some form of prism compensation may need to be provided for near vision. Such a compensation for vertical differential prism can be provided in several ways:

- Two separate pair of spectacles—one centred for distance vision and the second pair centred for near vision can be provided.
- Split design bifocals can be made where separate distance and reading lenses are cut in half and mounted together in a frame, each component being separately centred for distance and for near vision.
- A plano prism segment can be bonded to the lower half of the lens. For example – in the above example 2.4∆ base down prism might be bonded to the right lens to increase the prismatic effect at the right NVP to 4.8∆ base down which would match that of the left eye.

Different Prism at Distance and Near

There are occasions where different prisms are required at distance and near. These may be horizontal or vertical and require a different set of solutions. Refer to Chapter 10 for more detail.

Thinning Prism

Because of the decreasing radius of the front curve in the lower portion of an E-style bifocal or a progressive addition lens, the top of the lens ends up thicker than the bottom. Removing base up prism (work base down) will reduce the thickness at the top of the lens. The usual amount of thinning prism applied is 2/3rd of the near addition power. The benefit of thinning prism varies depending on the fitting position and the size of the frame. A progressive addition lens set low in the eye of a shallow frame will not benefit much from thinning prism but a progressive addition lens set high in a deeper aviator will definitely benefit because of this.

USES OF PRISM

Diagnostic Use of Prism

Prisms are used to assess the squint and heterophoria. Prism from the trial lens set and the prism bars are usually used for this purpose. These bars are composed of adjacent prisms of increasing power.

Therapeutic Use of Prism

The commonest therapeutic use of prisms in the orthoptics is in building up the fusional reserve of patients with convergence insufficiency. The base out prism is used during the patients exercise period. They are not worn constantly. Another therapeutic use of prism is to relieve diplopia in certain cases of squint. Prisms used in treatment include clip-on spectacle prisms for trial wear. An improvement on these is fresnel prism. Permanent incorporation of prism can be done in patients spectacles.

■ FRESNEL PRISM

In case of high prisms, the thick bases become cosmetically unappealing. An improvement on these is Fresnel prisms. A Fresnel prism consists of a plastic sheet of parallel tiny prisms of identical refracting angle **(Fig. 5.8)**. The overall prismatic effect is the same as that of a single large prism. Fresnel prisms are moulded from PVC (Polyvinyl chloride) to form a flexible sheet of prism. The sheet can be cut to the shape of the spectacle lens and fixed with the smooth side attached to the rear surface of the lens.

Functionally, Fresnel prisms reduce visual acuity and contrast sensitivity, particularly for prisms greater than 10Δ. The reductions in functions are mainly due to chromatic aberration, and are more pronounced for Fresnel prisms than for conventional prisms.

■ COMPOUNDING AND RESOLVING PRISMS

At times prescription calls for a vertical prism in conjunction with a horizontal prism, for example:

LE 3 Δ BD with 4Δ BO

The combined effect of above example could be produced by a single prism of appropriate power with its base in some oblique setting. To find this resultant

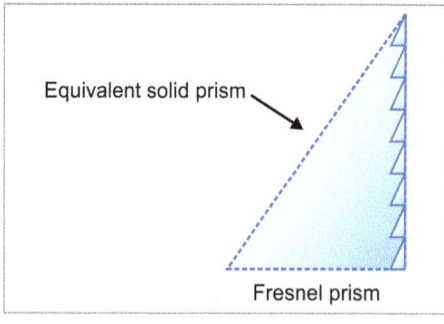

Fig. 5.8: Fresnel prism

prism, draw an accurate diagram. Remember standard notations, which say that the axis starts at zero on the right hand side of each eye and goes around anticlockwise from the observer's point of view **(Fig. 5.9)**.

Draw a set of lines at right angles to one another and mark the nasal area along with the primary directions based on this **(Fig. 5.10)**.

Picking a suitable scale, i.e., 1 cm = 1 diopter, mark a point equivalent to 3Δ down and 4Δ out **(Fig. 5.11)**.

Now construct a rectangle based on this and draws in a diagonal from the center of the cross lines to the corner of the rectangle as drawn in **Figure 5.12**.

This line represents both the magnitude and the base setting of the resultant prism. The line measures 5 units and therefore equals 5Δ diopters. The direction in relation to the center of the cross lines and nasal area is down and out. Expressed in terms of a 360° notation the base direction is 323°.

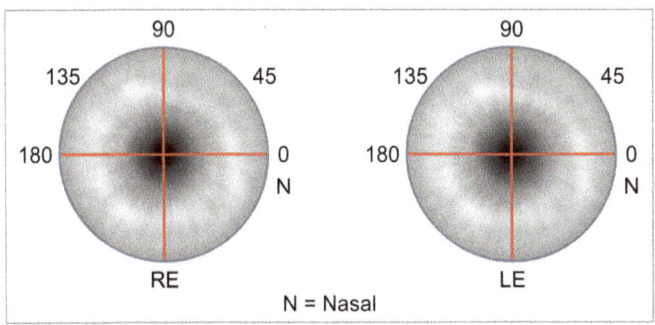

Fig. 5.9: Standard notation

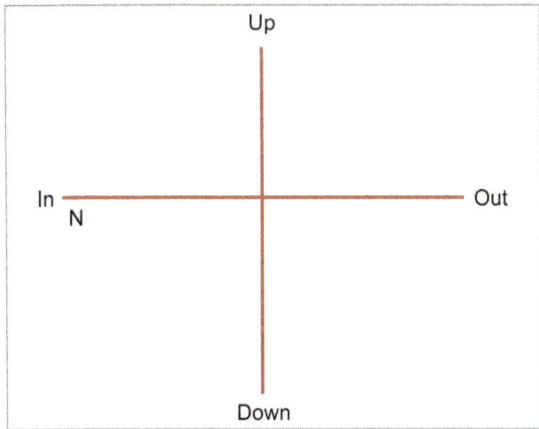

Fig. 5.10: Left eye representation showing principal directions

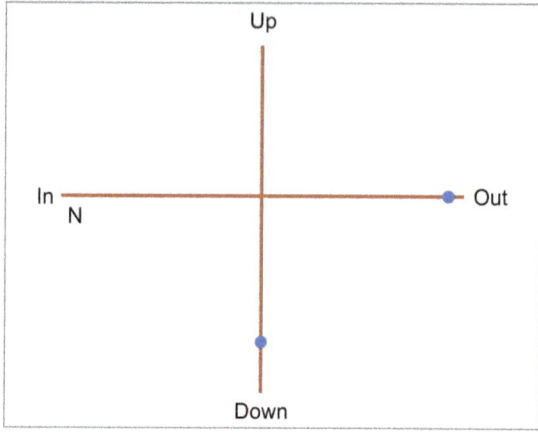

Fig. 5.11: Shows 3∆ down and 4∆ out to scale

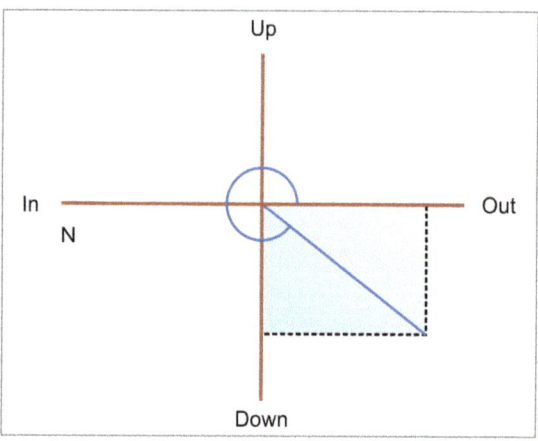

Fig. 5.12: Construction completed to show magnitude and angle of oblique prism

If a 180° notation is required the diagonal line needs to be extended so that it lies above the horizontal, measuring the axis indicated as shown in **Figure 5.13**. Therefore, the answer to compounding the prisms is:

5∆ base at 143° out

or, 5∆ base at 323°

There is a mathematical solution to compounding prisms. The formula is:

$$P_R = \sqrt{P_V^2 + P_H^2}$$

Where, P_R = Single resultant prism

P_V = Prism vertical

P_H = Prism horizontal

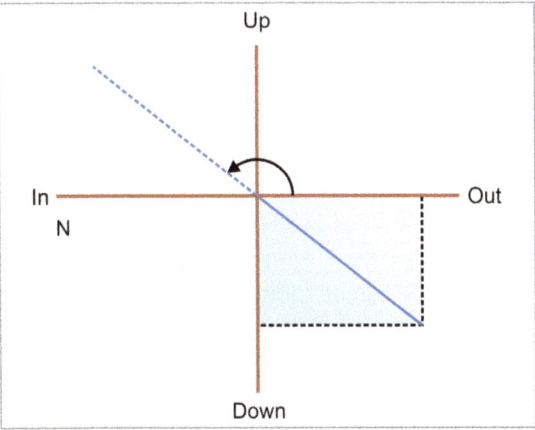

Fig. 5.13: Showing angle of prism in standard notation

Putting the values from the previous example:

PR = $\sqrt{3^2 + 4^2}$

PR = $\sqrt{9 + 16}$

PR = $\sqrt{25}$

PR = 5Δ

Now to obtain the base setting use:

$\tan \theta = \dfrac{P_V}{P_H}$

$\tan \theta = \dfrac{3}{4}$

$\tan \theta = 37°$

This needs to be converted to standard notation by subtracting from 180° (180 – 37 = 143).

Therefore, the answer is 143°.

PRISM AND LENS DECENTRATION

The general theory is if the lens power is 1.00 D and we decenter the lens by 10 mm, it produces 1Δ prism or if the lens power is 10.00 D and we decenter it by 1 mm, it also produces 1Δ prism. This is constant. The equation is:

(i) $d = \dfrac{10 \times P}{D}$

(ii) $P = \dfrac{D \times d}{10}$

Where, d = Decentration in mm
D = Dioptre or lens power
P = Prism degree

The required prism degree can be found out with the help of above equation. Now while grinding or surfacing, the lens prisms can be produced by keeping the edge difference for which the equation is:

Prism × Size of lens × 0.019 = Edge difference.

DETECTION OF PRISM IN AN OPTICAL LENS

Hold the glass up between the eye and an object which forms a straight line. If the continuity of the line in broken as seen in **Figure 5.14**, it implies that the prism is present and since the line appears to be deviated towards the apex, we know the direction of apex of the prism. The amount of displacement produced is the strength of the prism, and can be measured by neutralising. To do so put the prism lens of known strength in contact with the lens under checking with its apex in opposite direction. The prism lens with which the continuity of the lens is again established, represents the strength of the prism.

Lensometer can also be used to detect the prism dioptre. To check this get the best focus point of the target image and read the prismatic power. In most

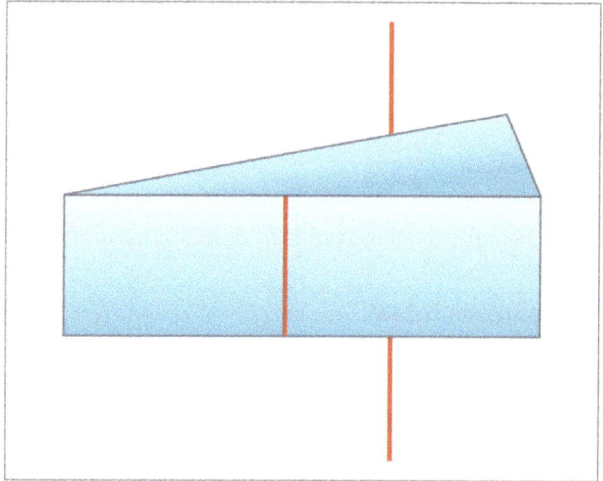

Fig. 5.14: Detecting prism in the lens

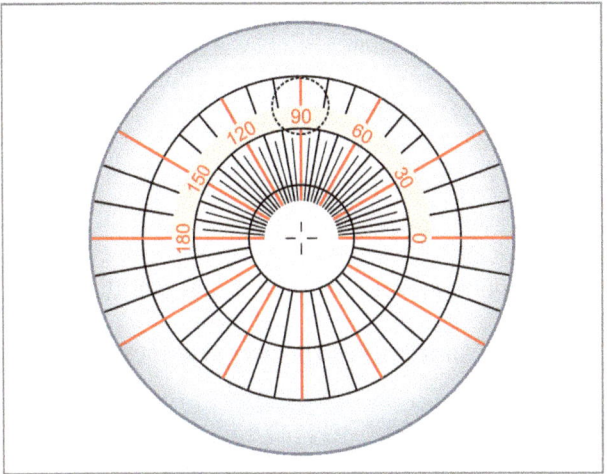

Fig. 5.15: Detection of prism in a lens using lensometer showing 2.5∆ prism

of the lensometer, each circle of the scale indicate one prism dioptre, as shown in the **Figure 5.15.** An additional accessory called 'prism compensator' is to be attached to the lensometer for higher dioptre of prism. **Figure 5.15** shows 2.5 prism dioptre towards 90° in PENTAX OLH-1 lensometer.

SUMMARY

The optics of ophthalmic prism is still nightmare to many optical students but in day-to-day practice, there is little complicated about them. Prisms, if used with care, can be used to improve the appearance of spectacles.

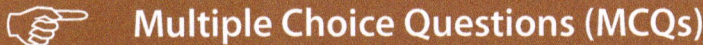

Multiple Choice Questions (MCQs)

1. The effect of prism on incident light:
    a. The emergent light is deviated towards the base of the prism
    b. The emergent light is deviated towards the apex of the prism
    c. There is a change in vergence of light
    d. None of the above

2. Which of the following is correct for the image formed by a prism?
    a. Image is minified
    b. Image is magnified
    c. Image is laterally inverted
    d. Image is deviated towards the apex

3. How is the angle of deviation of a prism determined?
   a. By the apical angle and refractive index of the prism material
   b. By the width of the base
   c. By the thickness of the prism
   d. All of the above

4. Which of the following is not true about prism?
   a. Prism deviates light towards its base
   b. Prism does not change the vergence of light
   c. The further the away from the optical center of the lens, greater is the prismatic effect
   d. The power of prism is described in terms of its focal length

Answers

1. a   2. d   3. a   4. d

Chapter 6

Lens Aberrations

Lens aberrations are defects that are caused when light rays from a point source pass through a correctly powered lens but fails to create a perfect image. When the eye views along the optical axis of the spectacle lens, image formed by the lens is not afflicted by any defects or aberrations. But in actual world, the eyes turn behind the lens to view through off-axis portion of the lens as shown in **Figures 6.1A to C,** it is then that the effect of lens aberration occurs. Lens aberrations defocus, degrade and deform the image quality. When the rays of light pass through the axial and paraxial portion of the lens, the lens behaves like a perfect optical system, imaging the point object as point image. Lens behavior through the peripheral portions is not like a perfect optical system.

Focal power of the lens is not accurate for the peripheral rays of light.

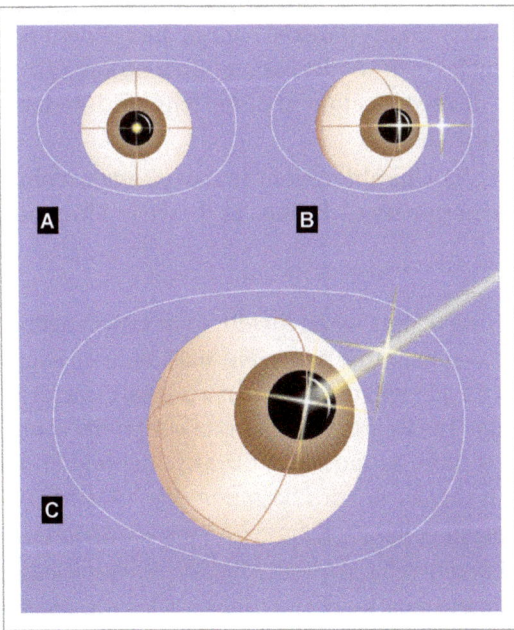

Figs 6.1A to C: Our eyes turn behind the lens to view through the off-axis. It is then the lens aberrations assume importance: (A) Primary direction; (B) Secondary direction; (C) Tertiary direction

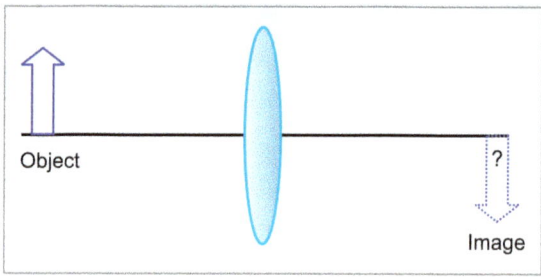

Fig. 6.2: Image quality is reduced

Flowchart 6.1: Types of lens aberrations

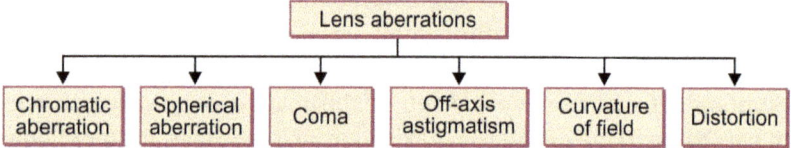

Lens aberrations are critical issues while designing ophthalmic lenses. Ideally, the off-axis performance of the lens should be the same as that of on-axis performance. But it is never so. The off-axis images are afflicted with various types of aberrations, which spoil the quality of image formed by the lens **(Fig. 6.2)**. Away from the paraxial region, the incident rays of light make larger and larger angles to the optical axis, and are no longer brought to a single point focus at the desired focal point of the lens, as described by the simple focal lens power formula.

There are six major lens aberrations that work against obtaining a perfect image through the periphery of the lens as shown in **Flowchart 6.1**.

■ CHROMATIC ABERRATION

Chromatic aberration occurs when the different wavelengths of light are not brought to the focus at the same point **(Fig. 6.3)**. Blue wavelength is refracted more than the red wavelength of light when it passes through a lens. The result is out of focus image. The wearer complains of peripheral color fringes around the object which is more pronounced off-axis. The higher the power of the lens—the greater is the chromatic aberration.

Chromatic aberration depends upon the material of the lens. Since the lens materials have a different refractive index for different wavelengths of light—the lens will have a different focal length for each wavelength. The refractive index is higher for shorter wavelength than the longer wavelength light, so focal length is less for shorter wavelength than that of the longer wavelength of light.

There are two types of chromatic aberration—axial or longitudinal chromatic aberration and lateral or transverse chromatic aberration. Axial chromatic

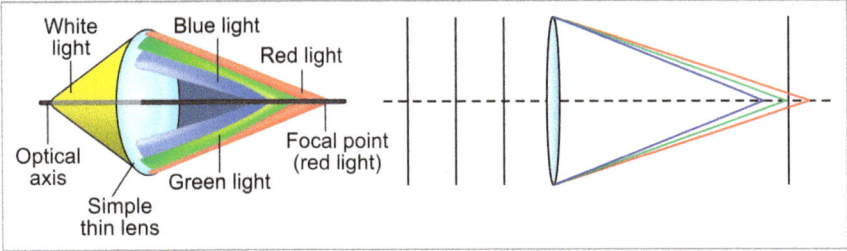

Fig. 6.3: Axial chromatic aberration

aberration occurs because of various focus points on the axis whereas lateral chromatic aberration is because of difference in magnifications.

Importance

Since chromatic aberration occurs because the refractive index of the lens material varies with the wavelength of the incident light, it gives rise to what is called the abbe value of the lens material which is denoted by V-value. Higher abbe value implies low chromatic aberrations and vice-versa. So polycarbonate lens with abbe value of 30 causes more chromatic aberration than CR39 lens with abbe value of 58.

Correction

- The easiest solution to minimize chromatic aberration is to change the lens material to higher abbe value.
- Careful placement of optical center with monocular pupillary distance and its height in a small frame may reduce the chromatic aberration.
- Reducing the vertex distance may also result in minimizing the effect of chromatic aberration.
- Anti-reflection coating with consumer education may also be tried to minimize the effect of chromatic aberration.
- The best solution is the achromatic lens system. The achromatic lens uses two different lens materials—one has a regular focal length and the other corrects the dispersion of the first lens **(Fig. 6.4)**. For this purpose, one lens is made of crown glass, i.e. low dispersion, while the other is made of flint glass, i.e. high dispersion. The crown lens concentrates on optical effect and introduces some dispersion and the flint glass aims at balancing this dispersion while having least possible optical influence on the lens function.

■ SPHERICAL ABERRATION

Spherical aberration is an axial and wide beam aberration **(Fig. 6.5)**. The light rays from the peripheral edge of the lens are refracted to a greater degree than the light rays passing through the center of the lens. Peripheral rays bend more

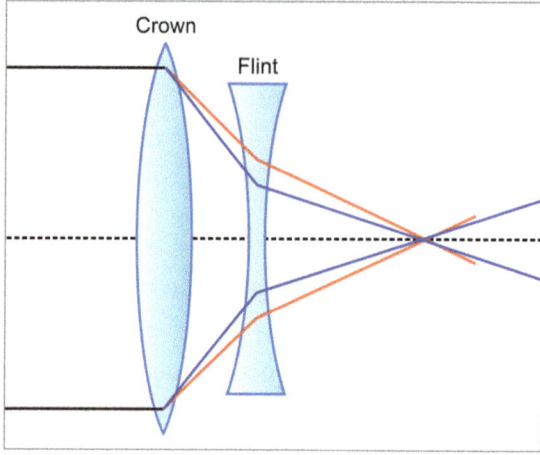

Fig. 6.4: Achromatic lens system

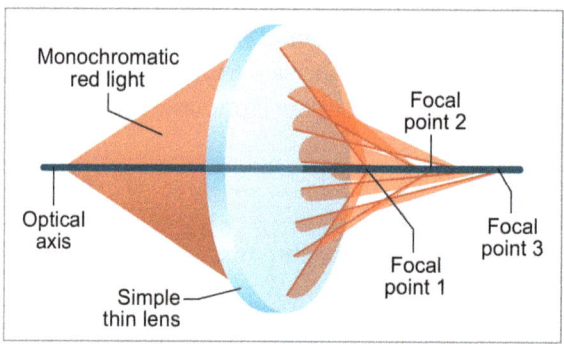

Fig 6.5: Spherical aberration

than the paraxial rays. Spherical aberration results in out of focus image and creates a slight blurring of the image that is minimized by the size of the lens.

Importance

Since spherical aberration is wide beam aberration, it is not very important in lens designing.

Correction

- Spherical aberration may be reduced by occluding the periphery of the lens such that only the paraxial zone is used.
- Lens form may also be adjusted to reduce spherical aberration. Aplanatic surface where periphery curve is less than the central curvature may be used.

OFF-AXIS ASTIGMATISM

Off-axis astigmatism or marginal astigmatism aberration is a small angle aberration. When a narrow beam of light enters obliquely to lens axis of a spherical lens, the refracted rays become astigmatic. The emerging rays, instead of uniting in a single image point, form two foci at right angles to one another with a disk of least confusion **(Fig. 6.6)**. On joining the two foci, a line image is created. The plane containing the optical axis of the surface is referred to as the "tangential plane" and the plane at the right angle to the tangential plane is referred to as the "sagittal plane". Another way to understand the effect of off-axis astigmatism is—tilting a spherical lens adds spherical and cylinder of the same sign as the original lens and is called astigmatism of oblique incidence. The effect of off-axis astigmatism is that it produces blurring of image due to imposition of unwanted spherical–cylinder between the lens and the eye. It also reduces contrast, and as the aperture is opened wider and wider, the astigmatic figure of off-axis astigmatic aberration becomes the typical cometic figure.

Importance

Since off-axis astigmatism is a small angle aberration, it is very important in ophthalmic lens designing. It is the aberration modern corrected curve design seeks to eliminate.

Correction

It is considerably affected by the form of the lens used. It is much worse in bi- convex and bi-concave lens than meniscus lens form. It may be reduced by the use of an aspheric surface or by a suitable choice of lens bending, i.e. by using corrected curve theory. Proper use of pantoscopic tilt with optical center height may help reducing off-axis astigmatism.

> Off-axis astigmatism is the aberration modern corrected curve design seeks to eliminate

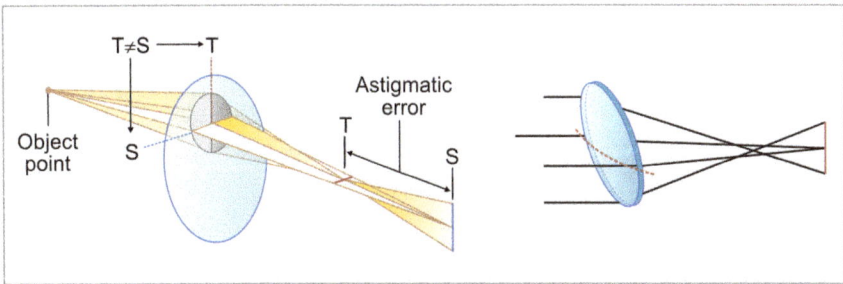

Fig. 6.6: Light rays entering obliquely to lens axis of a spherical lens, the refracted rays become astigmatic

COMA

Coma is a wide beam aberration. It is applied to oblique rays coming from points not lying on the principal axis. Oblique rays passing through the periphery of the lens are deviated more than the central rays and come to focus near the principal axis. The result is unequal magnification of the image formed by the different zones of the lens. The composite image is not circular, but elongated like a comet **(Fig. 6.7)**.

Coma is associated with the off-axis object points. It occurs because magnification is the function of the height of the rays of the light. It is the worst type of aberration as it degrades and deforms the image of a point object. The funny part is that a lens with considerable coma may produce a sharp image at the center of the field, but becomes increasingly blurred towards the edges.

Correction

The effect of cometic aberration can be minimized by using parabolic curves. Aspheric lens design helps reduce coma in high plus power.

CURVATURE OF FIELD

Curvature of field is a phenomenon which causes the image formation of a plane to become curved like the inside of a shallow bowl, preventing the lens from producing a flat image of a flat object **(Fig. 6.8)**. This may occur even when the spherical aberration, off-axis astigmatism and coma have been eliminated. The effect is largely dependent upon the refractive index of the lens material and the curvature of the lens surface.

This causes an unequal vertex distance between the center of the lens surface and its periphery. So the image so focused is either sharp on the edges or in the center. When the center of the image is in focus, the periphery is out of focus and when the periphery is in focus, the center is out of focus.

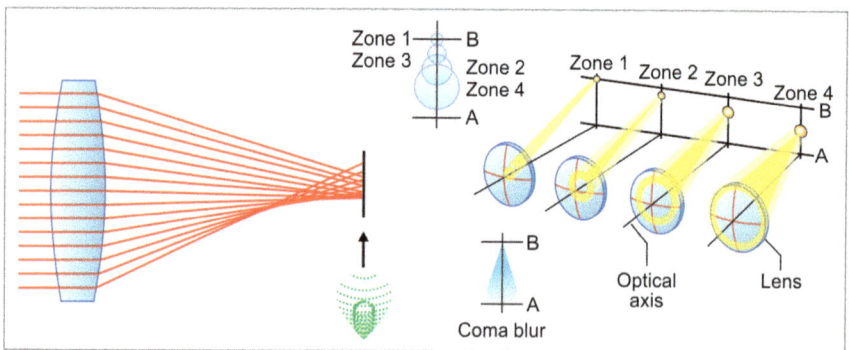

Fig. 6.7: Peripheral rays form larger image than paraxial rays

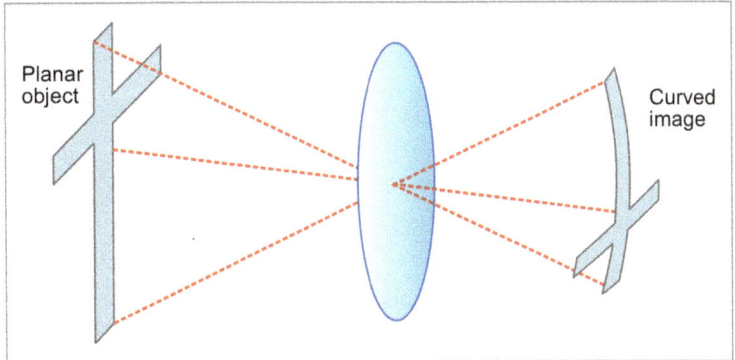

Fig. 6.8: Light focused through a curved lens forms a curved image

Curvature of field is of great concern for optical devices that require a flat image plane, such as cameras.

Correction

Curvature of field affects peripheral vision. Curvature of field is minimized with corrected curve design base curvatures. As a rule, if off-axis astigmatic aberration is corrected, the effect of curvature of field is also reduced. Far-point sphere in human eye is also curved, that compensates to some extent.

DISTORTION

Distortion is another aberration of thick lenses. Distortion of image may be observed even when the object is sharply imaged. It is characterized by deshaping of image **(Fig 6.9)**. There are two types of distortions resulting from lateral magnification of the image that results in a lateral displacement of the image.

Barrel Distortion

Barrel distortion is produced in minus power lens where the rays in the center are more magnified than the rays farther off-axis. This is due to minification of corners of a square grid more from minus lens.

Pincushion Distortion

Pincushion effect is produced in plus lens where the central rays are less magnified. This is due to the magnification of corners of a square object more from plus lens. Distortion is of minor importance in ophthalmic lens designing. It is a problem mainly of high power lens. It can be minimized by using steep back surface.

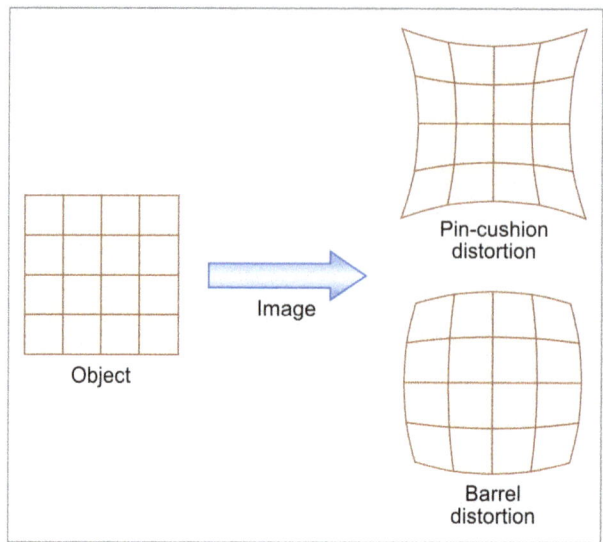

Fig. 6.9: Pin cushion with plus lens and barrel distortion with minus lens

The entire discussion may be summarized as given in **Table 6.1**.

Lens aberrations are important considerations while lens designing as they are inherent to lenses. For various reasons and also because of limitations of optics not all aberrations can be controlled. The truth is all aberrations occur together. It is difficult to understand the exact effect of each individual aberration. The wide angle spherical and cometic aberrations are of no importance since the entrance pupil of the eye is so small. The visual system adapts quickly to distortion, so the additional aberration of spectacle lens may be ignored. Thus the spectacle lens designer is left only with the job of correcting astigmatism and curvature of field within tolerable limits so as to produce maximum dynamic field of vision for the patients.

Table 6.1: Summarization of lens aberrations

Aberration	Direction of aberration	Type of aberration	Type and location of object
Spherical aberration	Longitudinal	Wide beam aberration	On and off-axis aberration
Coma	Transverse	Wide beam aberration	Off-axis aberration
Off-axis astigmatism	Longitudinal	Narrow beam aberration	Off-axis aberration
Curvature of field	Longitudinal	Curvature	Extended objects
Distortion	Transverse	Shape distortion	Extended objects

Multiple Choice Questions (MCQs)

1. Pincushion distortion is produced by:
   a. Minus power
   b. Plus power
   c. Prism
   d. All of the above

2. Barrel distortion is produced by:
   a. Minus power
   b. Plus power
   c. Prism
   d. All of the above

3. Which of the following is not a wide beam aberration?
   a. Spherical aberration
   b. Coma
   c. Off-axis astigmatism
   d. None of the above

4. Which of the following type of aberration is not very important while designing a spectacle lens?
   a. Spherical aberration
   b. Off-axis aberration
   c. Distortion
   d. Curvature of field

5. Which of the following lens aberration occur more because of lens material than because of lens design?
   a. Spherical aberration
   b. Comatic aberration
   c. Marginal astigmatism
   d. Chromatic aberration

6. Which of the following is true about chromatic aberration?
   a. It results from the dispersive power of the lens material
   b. It depends on the refractive index of the lens material
   c. It occurs with light of same wavelength
   d. It depends on the refractive power of the lens

7. The comatic aberration is found in image of a point object situated:
   a. On the axis
   b. Off the axis
   c. Far off the axis
   d. None of the above

8. The spherical aberration arises due to the fact that:
   a. The different zones of the lens have different magnification
   b. The different zones of the lens have different focal lengths
   c. The different zones of the lens have different diameter
   d. The different zones of the lens have different frequencies.

9. The inability of a lens to form the point image of a point object situated off the axis is called:
   a. Spherical aberration
   b. Comatic aberration
   c. Chromatic aberration
   d. Astigmatism

Answers

1. b   2. a   3. c   4. a   5. d   6. a   7. b   8. b   9. b

Chapter 7

Tinted Lens

THE ELECTROMAGNETIC SPECTRUM

The electromagnetic spectrum is the gamut of radiations which include cosmic rays, gamma rays, x-rays, ultraviolet rays, visible light, infrared rays, radio waves and so on **(Fig. 7.1)**. Light is measured by its wavelength (in nanometers) or frequency (in Hertz). One wavelength. equals the distance between two successive wave crests or troughs **(Fig. 7.2)**. The above classification is based on their wavelengths. The classification is based on their wavelengths. In ophthalmic optics, we are concerned with a relatively narrow band of the electro-magnetic spectrum. The wavelengths in this region are extremely short and are expressed in nanometers (nm). This is the unit of wavelength and is one thousand millionth part of a meter or one millionth part of a millimeter.

The visible spectrum gives rise to the sensation of light. It extends from about 380 nm to 780 nm. Various wavebands within this region are associated with different color sensations **(Fig. 7.3)**. For example, a light of 650 nm gives rise to the sensation of red, 480 nm describes a blue light, and 580 nm describes a light having yellow hue.

The radiations emitted by most sources of light and heat, whether natural or artificial, not only include all the wavelengths of the visible spectrum but also extend into the neighboring region, i.e., the ultraviolet and infrared. Although,

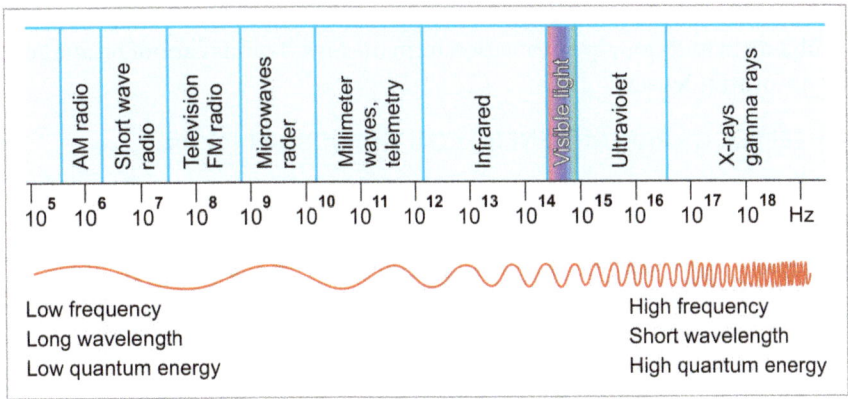

Fig. 7.1: Electromagnetic spectrum

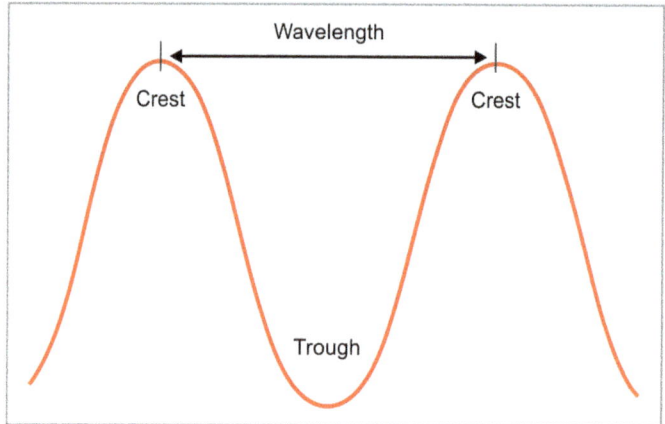

Fig. 7.2: Wavelength is the distance between one wave crest to the next

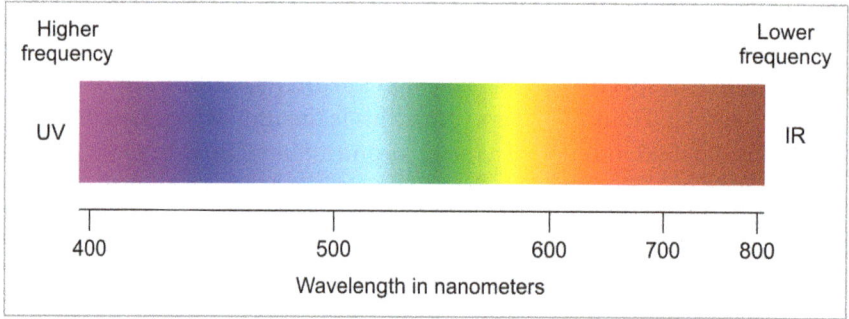

Fig. 7.3: Visible spectrum

not perceived as light, these radiations are capable of doing serious damage to the eyes, if they are of sufficient intensity. Other radiations such as X-rays, gamma rays are also damaging to the eyes. But since they are also damaging to the other bodily functions, they are not treated solely as an ophthalmic problem. In addition, eye protection from these radiations cannot be attained by absorptive lenses.

EFFECT OF RADIANT ENERGY ON THE OCULAR TISSUES

Radiation is characterized by its wavelength. The portion of the total spectrum which is of primary ophthalmic concern is usually divided into ultraviolet, the visible and the infrared. Other radiations such as X-ray, gamma ray and many other forms of nuclear radiations are also damaging to the eyes. But since they are also damaging to the other bodily functions, they are not treated as solely an ophthalmic problem.

The visible spectrum: The media of the eye is transparent throughout the visible spectrum which may be taken as existing between 380 nm to 780 nm.

Within this region the energy is transmitted to excite the sensation of the vision and has no harmful effects upon the tissues under the ordinary intensities of radiation. In recent years, concern has been expressed over the potential effects of short-wave visible radiation on ocular tissues. The blue light hazard remains a controversial topic and, at present, it is suggested in the appropriate literature that under normal circumstances not much of the risk is expected.

Infrared: The region above 780 nm is referred to as the infrared end of the spectrum. The effect of radiant energy from the infrared region, depending upon the intensity and degree of duration, has a thermal effect. Of the total incident infrared radiant energy on the eye, 97% is absorbed by the cornea, iris, lens and vitreous and the remaining 3% reaches the retina. Therefore, the thermal effect of long-wave radiation can involve all the tissues of the eyes, depending upon the degree of concentration of energy.

Ultraviolet: Extending from 380 nm into the lower regions of the spectrum, ultraviolet energy absorption commences and has an abiotic effect. Abiotic action produces chemical changes in the cornea and lens affecting the protein in the cells. The extent of tissue injury depends on the intensity of the energy reaching the tissue and time of exposure.

The chief natural source of UV rays is the sun. Artificial sources of UV include incandescent light, gas discharge, low pressure mercury, xenon lamps, etc.

For convenience, UV radiation is subdivided into three groups **(Fig. 7.4)**:
1. **UVC:** It has the shortest wavelengths from 200 nm to 290 nm and is, therefore, potentially the most harmful to us because the shorter wavelengths always have the highest energy. When this high energy is transferred to human tissue, it can be damaging, especially with repeated exposures. Fortunately the ozone layer of the earth screens it out.
2. **UVB:** Wavelength between 290 nm to 320 nm are responsible for sunburns and snow blindness. The amount of ultraviolet affecting a person is

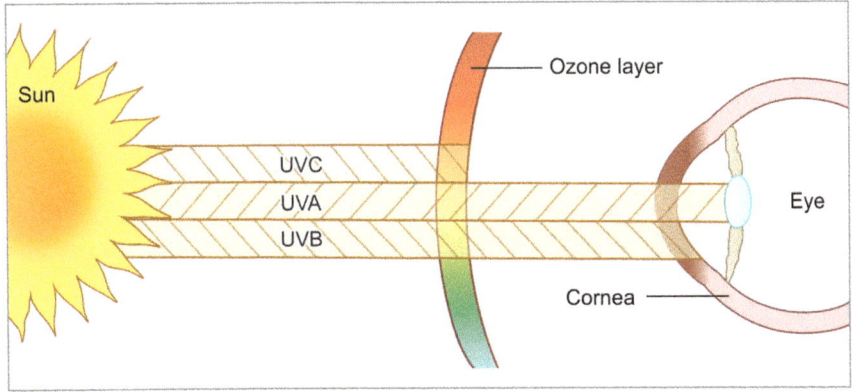

Fig. 7.4: Components of UV light

substantially increased by reflection from surfaces such as snow, sand, concrete and water.

3. **UVA:** Wavelengths between 320 nm to 380 nm is possibly the cause of most concern for the ophthalmic professionals, as it enters the eyes, causing chronic damage to the eye.

It is, therefore, necessary to protect the ocular tissue as much as possible from the effect of UV rays. The cornea absorbs UV radiation below 300 nm. It is susceptible to ultraviolet related problems such as pterygium, snow blindness and photokeratitis. The eyes crystalline lens takes in UV and injures itself. Over years of absorption and exposure, the lens may become yellow or brown, indicating the need for cataract surgery.

ABSORPTION CHARACTERISTICS OF CONVENTIONAL CROWN GLASS

When light is incident on ophthalmic crown lens, some of the light is reflected, some is absorbed and the remainder is transmitted. The percentage of light that is lost by reflection from each surface can be determined by Fresnel's law, assuming normal incident light:

$$(n - 1 / n + 1)^2$$

Where n = index of refraction of the lens.

For crown glass having an index of refraction of 1.523, the reflection factor would be:

$$(1.523 - 1 / 1.523 + 1)^2 = 0.043 \text{ or } 4.3\%$$

The amount of light lost by reflection from the front and back surfaces, therefore would be:

$$2 \times 4.3 = 8.6\%$$

Since the refractive index varies with the wavelength, the surface reflectance varies accordingly. It is the highest at the blue end of the spectrum.

The amount of light lost by absorption, for crown glass, is less than 1% per centimeter of lens thickness. Therefore, for a lens of 0.2 cm thick, loss by absorption would be approximately 0.2%. The transmission for this lens would be:

$$100\% - (8.6\% + 0.2\%) = 91.2\%$$

The crown glass absorbs all the UV light below 290 nm. But unfortunately, it is the UV rays between 290 nm and 380 nm as noted previously, are more disturbing. Infrared rays are transmitted in the same proportion as are visible rays.

FILTER LENSES

The tinted lenses are also called filters. The filters selectively absorb some colors and reflect or transmit others. The question that is often asked is 'How does a tinted lens create or alter color, when it is essentially acting as a filter which blocks light? The answer lies in the fact that to create one color in the spectrum, it destroys the "complementary color". The easiest way to understand the meaning of complementary colors is to take the reference of color wheel as shown in **Figure 7.5**. Colors that lie opposite to each other on the color wheel are considered to be complementary colors. This can also be explained with an example. A lens containing special tint molecules to absorb blue light, will allow the other colors of the spectrum to pass through and will create a lens with a yellow appearance. The body will have the same color of the part of the spectrum in which it is placed. The second important question is 'Where does the blue light go?' Since energy cannot be destroyed, it ends up being converted into heat energy by the tint molecules. An alternative to absorption is to reflect light, a method adopted in mirror coatings. The same complementary color theory applies, so that a "blue" mirror reflects yellow light.

In order to obtain specific color, appropriate metals and metal oxides are added to glass during its manufacturing process to change its color, thereby altering the absorption deliberately in almost any desired way, both within and beyond the visible spectrum. Besides, some oxides like titanium is used to intensify and brighten other glass colorants. The way the glass is heated and cooled can also significantly affect the colors produced by these compounds. The chemistry involved is complex and needs in depth study for clear understanding.

Grey: Grey filter is the most popular protection tint. It has an even transmission through the whole visible spectrum. So this is a neutral density filter. This

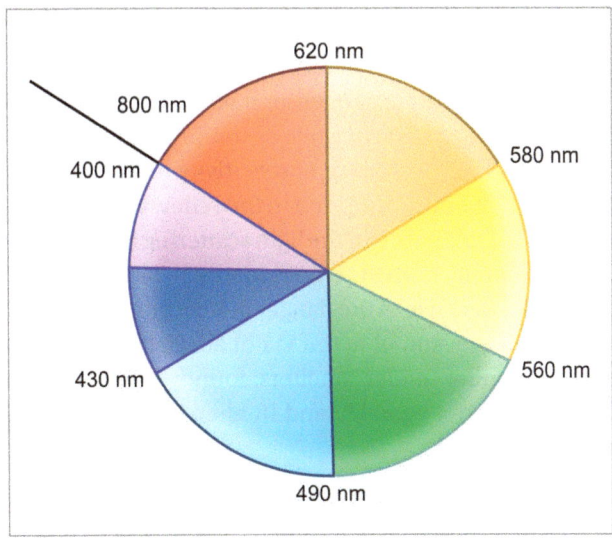

Fig. 7.5: Color wheel

characteristic allows colors to be seen in their natural state relative to one another without destroying them. It does reduce the intensity, but does not block any particular wavelength. As they reduce the amount of all light colors transmitted to the eye, dark grey filters may reduce visual acuity slightly. By reducing the total amount of light entering the eye on very bright days, the brightness can be adjusted to give a clearer sight picture which can compensate for any loss in visual acuity compared to not using a filter. So it is likely to be favored by the light sensitive patients. Those who can not tolerate color distortion or whose job requires accurate color discrimination, also favor grey tint. Grey lenses offer good protection against glare, making them a good choice for driving and general use. Because it absorbs light equally over the whole visible spectrum, it is not the best contrast enhancing color.

Yellow: Chromium or sulphur oxides are used to give rise to yellow tint filter. Uranium oxides can also be used for the same purpose. Yellow filters absorb blue, violet and UV light while allowing a larger percentage of other frequencies through. Since blue light tends to bounce and scatter, it can create a kind of glare known as blue haze, thereby reducing the contrast. The yellow tint virtually eliminates the blue/UV end of the spectrum and has the effect of making everything bright and sharp. The tint concentrates light in the area of the spectrum to which the eye is most sensitive. If an individual is already light sensitive then the experience is heightened looking through a yellow or orange filter. Someone who is not light sensitive would really appreciate the contrast enhancing effect of yellow filter. That is why yellow filter is likely to be favored in visually demanding sports like trap shooting and snow skiing, especially on overcast days. This tint really distorts color perception, which makes it inappropriate for any activity that relies on accurate color perception.

Blue: Small concentration of cobalt (0.025% to 0.1%) yield blue glass. Blue filter glass is likely to transmit more dangerous high energy part of the spectrum, i.e. shorter wavelengths blue and UV while absorbing the light into the yellow and orange wavelengths. The eyes lack of sensitivity to this part of the spectrum adds to the danger. But the absorption in the yellow wavelength makes it good for light sensitive individuals. But the light scattering effect of the blue light out weighs the relief they get from the elimination of peak sensitivity wavelength of yellow and orange. Because of the danger of high energy blue light intensified by the brilliance of the sun, blue tint is not advisable for outdoor use. It can be prescribed for boiler tender, smelters, foundry work and certain types of furnace work. As it is not good UV and IR filter, it is not intended for welding application.

Green: The green tinted glass lens obtains its color and characteristic transmission curve from ferrous oxide metal. Green filters transmit wavelengths of around 500 nm, i.e., green as well as yellow, orange and at the higher end red while absorbing some, but not all of the blue-violet region. It has a good UV as well as infrared heat absorbing properties. It makes a very good sunglass tint because of its contrast enhancing properties. It allows true color perception and real protection in bright light. It reduces eyestrain in bright light and also glare. It is a good intermediate filter to use when grey or yellow does not seem right.

Red: Red filter gets its color characteristics because of higher concentration of selenium. Red filter strongly blocks the transmission of blue and blue-green wavelengths, resulting in very sharply defined contrast. It allows excellent depth perception in low light, and is good for skiing and hunting. Red tint can be helpful for hue discrimination in color deficiency. This effect might be enhanced by relating the tint to the anomaly, a red tint for protanopes and a green for deuteranopes. It is also possible that the choice will not be as simple as this or the reverse or that the greatest effect is achieved by another color or different color in each eye.

Pink: Pink is an example of unsaturated red. Cerium is added to the batch mix to give rise to pinkish tint. Psychologically pink has been judged as the "sweetest" color. They are prescribed mainly to attenuate the light in a pleasing way. They have the absorption properties in the UV and blue light region. Pink may be the color of choice when there is some neurological problem.

Amber: Amber is fluorescent that increases the contrast of the objects so that every cracks and curbs stand out in our field of vision. Non-metallic element sulphur is used with iron to produce amber glass, the color of which can vary from very light straw to deep reddish brown. Night vision with amber tint brightens the darkness in front of a vehicle so that the subject can see more details. In addition, the amber tint also reduces the glare from front headlights. Amber is more of a selective filter. It also offers excellent light management properties on cloudy or rainy days. Therefore, it is great for lower light conditions like – golf, shooting, fishing, skiing etc. This "light enhancing effect" reduces the eye strain. It also improves visual acuity and depth perception.

Brown: Brown tints are good general purpose filters. They have added benefit of reducing glare and molecules that mainly absorbs total UV light below 400nm. In the visible region of spectrum, transmission is controlled with high peaks in the blue, green and red region, resulting in a color enhancing effect. It is an excellent contrast enhancing filter and is very much suitable for sun protection. Brown is an ideal tint for drivers for day time driving as it has three effects - eliminates the "blue blur" substantially, increases the contrast and gives the wearer an impression of higher light transmission.

Orange: In normal use, orange is the essence of brown, so a tint diagnosis of orange would transmit to a brown tint. Orange filter allows transmission of light that is the same color as the filter and promote tonal separation in that color. They tend to reduce the transmission of blue and green wavelength, thus increasing the contrast. So the image appears sharper. It is an ideal support for cycling, mountain tours, skiing and a lot more.

Violet: Violet is the least chosen tint of all. It is almost as photoactive as ultraviolet and can irritate eyes and even cause eye damage.

METHODS OF LENS TINTING

A spectacle lens is said to be tinted if the transmission of light is deliberately decreased by any means, either over the whole of the visible spectrum and its neighbouring regions, or merely a part of it. They offer selective absorption for each wavelengths of the spectrum, and this determines their tints. Such absorption may be fixed or variable. Fixed absorption is the case with all traditional fixed tinted glasses, whereas, photochromic glasses offer variable absorption where transparency varies according to light conditions.

Color results from the absorbent properties of glasses in the visible spectrum. The body will have the color of the part of the spectrum in which it is placed.

Tinted lenses should not alter the colors of objects viewed through them and force the eye into constant efforts of adaptation. However, colors sometimes happen to be inspired by fashion, especially when it comes to sunglasses. To ascertain the real properties of tinted lenses, we have to refer to their transmittance curves which show the percentage of light transmitted in the different zones of the spectrum and reveal the absorbent properties of the lens.

Spectacle lenses may be tinted in two different ways as shown by **Flowchart 7.1**.

Integral Tints

Integral tint has been the only method by which a glass lens could be tinted for several years. Various metallic oxides were added to the batch materials

Flowchart 7.1: Types of tinted lens

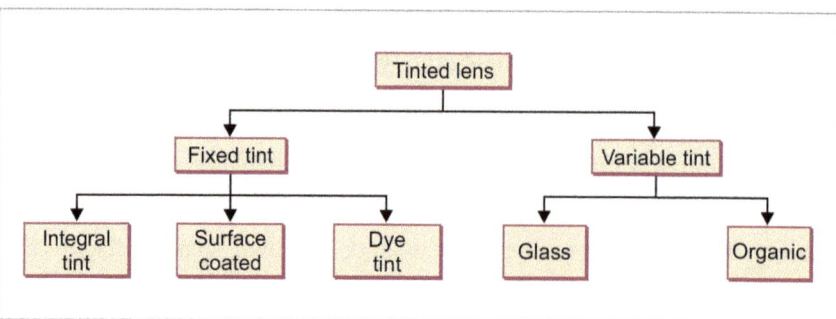

to give the lens a specific color. For example, cerium oxide was added to the batch mix to give rise to pinkish tint while cobalt oxide was added to create blue tint lenses. Nickel oxide gives rise to brown tints. Numerous Rare Earths like neodymium , erbium were also used. Adding these oxides lead to selective absorption for each wavelength in the spectrum, and thus determine the tint.

Light passing through a homogeneous material suffers a continuous loss by absorption. The loss can be understood by imaging the lens or filter to be made up of a number of very thin layers, each of which absorbs a constant proportion of the radiant energy emerging from the previous layer. This proportion is not necessarily the same for all wavelengths. By adding the various metallic oxides or other compounds to the glass constituents, the absorption can be deliberately increased in almost any desired way, both within and beyond the visible spectrum. If the absorption is uniform within the visible spectrum, the tint imparted to the material will be grey or neutral. Selective absorption gives rise to a definitive hue. Thus, a relatively higher absorption in the red region of the spectrum would produce a greenish tint.

The effect of thickness can be seen as a variation in transmission across the lens. Normally, absorptive lenses are rated in terms of transmission for a lens of a constant thickness of 2 mm. However, actual transmission may differ at various points on a lens of high power. In addition, it may also lead to uneven density of tint across the lens which may be cosmetically unattractive. Accordingly, high plus lens will have lower actual transmission and higher density of tint at the center of the lens as compare to high minus lens which will show lower density of tint at the center and higher actual transmission. For lenses having cylindrical component, the two principal meridians will behave differently.

The integral tinted or solid tinted glasses have disappeared from the optical industry because of several reasons as mentioned below:
- Huge number of lenses were to be produced in different base curves, different tints, different lens diameter and different additions which resulted in large inventory and logistic cost for the manufacturer.
- The disadvantages of different densities of tints from center to edge was cosmetically unacceptable.
- A possibility of mismatch of tints for different lens prescription between right and left lenses.

Surface Tinting/Coating

An absorptive coating may be applied to a clear glass lens through the use of metallic oxide applied to the lens in a vacuum. There are several advantages of such coatings. First, they are uniform in density regardless of the lens prescription to which they are applied. Color coated lenses have a predictable transmission, whereas solid tinted lenses which exhibit a darker tint as the glass thickens, transmission curve varies across the surface. Color coated lenses do not have such problems. In addition, they are available in a wide range of colors and transmission. Color coatings may be removed and the lens may be recoated to give the effect of new color. One drawback of the color coated lenses is that they must be cared for in a manner similar to that used for plastic lenses.

Transmission curves for color coated lenses are generally more even across the spectrum than either glass with integral tinting or dyed plastic. Surface coating may be possible in the following ways:

1. Mirror coating: A mirror coating can be applied by a vacuum process to the front surface of the lens causing the lens to have the same properties as a two way mirror. The observer, unable to see the wearer's eyes, sees his own image reflected from the lens. The wearer is able to look through the lens normally. There is, of course, a reduction in the transmission of the lens simply because of the high percentage of light reflected. Mirror coatings are often used in combination with a tinted lens to provide more protection from intense sunlight. Mirror coating may be full, i.e. uniform throughout the lens surface or it may be graduated. The process is also capable of obtaining a whole variety of effects, i.e. a range of colors and mirrors, which is for reasons of fashion are highly popular in sunglasses. In case of lens having thick edges, only edge coating is also possible for cosmetic improvement. Edge coating is the application of the color that matches the frame to the bevel area of the lens, camouflaging the edge. The purpose of such a process is to rid the lenses of the concentric rings visible to the observer. These rings accentuate the effect of the thick glasses. But it should be done very cautiously with a laboratory expert in this area. Mirror coated lenses work by reflecting back specific wavelengths, whereas solid tints work by absorbing the wavelengths or light energy. Light energy so absorbed expresses itself in the form of heat which might irradiate the eyes. But this does not occur in case of vacuum tints as the energy is reflected away. The wearer also gets the benefits because the depth of the tint is uniform over the whole lens area, whatever the power and the thickness of the lens. The prescription house benefits because it minimizes the necessity for keeping stocks of necessary blanks.

2. Dye tinting: Resin lenses can be tinted by immersing in a container of dye. The container is put in a unit that allows heat to be transferred to the dye. The longer the lenses remain in the dye, the more dye will be absorbed. Thus making them darker. The dye penetrates the lens material and becomes the part of it. It can not be rubbed off. Red, yellow and blue are the three primary dyes with which almost all other colors can be made. For example, blue and yellow can be mixed together to make green.

The dye can be purchased either in powder or liquid form which are then mixed with previously boiled water. The concentrate so prepared is brought up to a temperature of 92 to 96°C and a pair of lens is immersed together to have the similar tint. Interesting tint combination can be created to an individuals imagination. Graduated and double graduated effects are comparatively easy to achieve with the aid of a pulley mechanism which gradually lifts the lenses out of the tint tank, thus imparting more tint on one part of the lens than the others.

One thing must be kept in the mind that it is difficult to predict how a pair of lens will react when immersed into a tint bath. Even though both the lens may be of the same material and also from the same manufacturer, the "take up" rate between the right and the left lens may be different. This can be due to a number of factors. One reason could be that one lens has been in storage for longer period than the other and thereby react differently when immersed into the tint bath. To reduce such problems always try to ensure that same manufacturer's lenses are tinted together and both the lenses must be of the same index because higher index resin materials exhibit different characteristics that prevent them from being tinted to the darker shades.

The dye tints are absorbed into both surfaces equally; they are not affected by the power of the lens and will therefore have an even tint regardless of prescription.

PHOTOCHROMIC LENSES

Photochromic lenses are lenses that visibly darken and fade indefinitely under bright and dull light respectively. They were developed by Dr WH Armistead and SD Stookey at Corning Incorporated in 1964. A photochromic glass lens contains billions of microscopic crystals of Silver Halide. When exposed to direct sunlight or UV light, these crystals absorb energy and cause the formation of metallic silver deposit on silver halide crystals **(Fig. 7.6)**. It is this metallic silver that absorbs the light. This reduces the amount of light passing through the lens and the lens turns darker. With the disappearance of UV rays or sunlight, the lens returns to its faded state by the reconvertion of deposited metallic silver into silver halide. Since these crystals are within the lens material, the process of darkening and fading can be repeated.

FACTORS AFFECTING PHOTOCHROMATISM

Although, exposure to ultraviolet light is one of the conditions that influence photo chromic lens transmission most, several other factors also contribute to lighting and darkening phenomenon. They are somewhat temperature dependent. Assuming the same degree of illumination, they will be darker when it is colder and lighter more than when it is warmer. This is slightly ironic as of course they are looked upon as a sunglass lens to be used in warm conditions. Because they react more in colder climates, there are some photochromic lenses where the manufacturer uses a warning stating that they should not be worn in freezing or cold conditions as the lens would darken to virtually zero transmission.

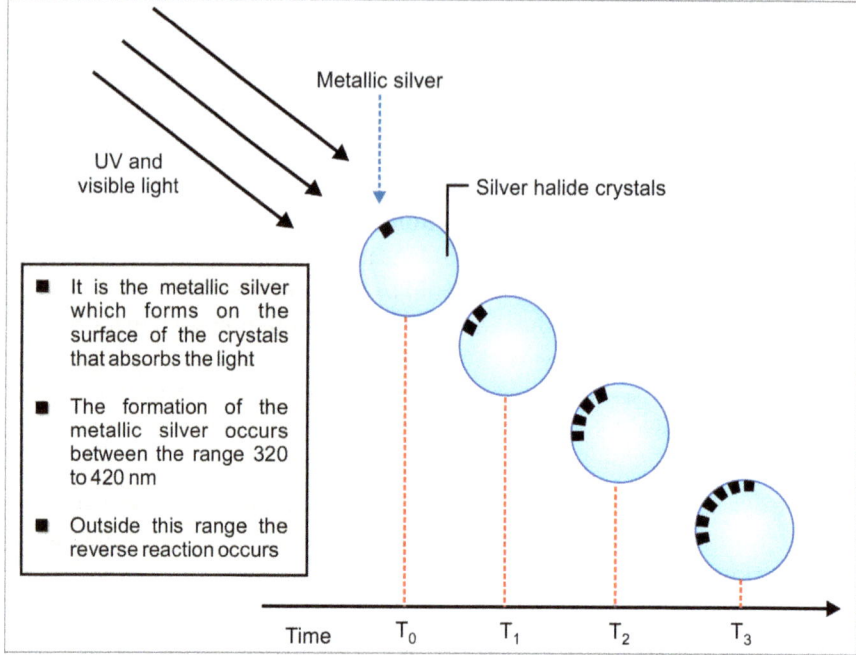

Fig. 7.6: Darkening process of photochromatic lens

Lens thickness has an effect on the density of the tint. The silver halides run evenly through the lens, and therefore the thicker the lens, the more of them is there to absorb the light, hence the tint would be darker. Care must be exercised when looking at transmission graphs or curves put out by the various photochromic lens manufacturers. They are all usually based on 2 mm thick sample at a specific stated temperature. Any variance in these values will affect the transmission characteristics.

Photochromic lenses achieve their full changing range and speed only after a "break - in" period, i.e., they tend to improve with age. The more light/dark cycles that they go through, the better they perform. It is, therefore, very common for patients supplied with a new pair of photochromic lens to complain that they do not change as good as their old pair. Because of the above it is recommended that these lenses are always replaced in pairs to ensure best possible tint match. Photochromic performance slows down if the lenses are not exposed to radiations for a longer period of time and when they are re-exposed the performance returns to normal.

TINT OPTIONS IN PHOTOCHROMIC LENSES

Glass photochromic lens usually come in two basic colors—grey and brown **(Fig 7.7)**. Technically it is possible to obtain other tint also, but demand has to be sufficient to justify the production of the particular tint. It has been

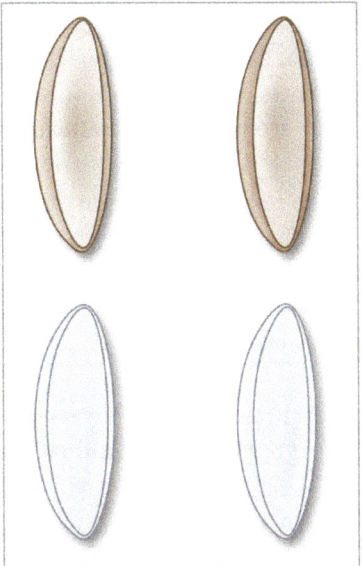

Fig. 7.7: Photochromatic lenses—grey and brown

attempted in the past to make pink and green photochromic lens, but it seems to have settled down to a choice between grey and brown.

RESIN PHOTOCHROMIC LENS

Photochromic resin lenses utilize a significantly different photochromic technology than that is used for glass. Photochromic compounds can be incorporated into a resin lens by applying either a photochromatic coating or dye to the lens or by penetration of the surface, known as imbibitions. Using the imbibing technique it is possible to provide a uniform distribution of millions of photosensitive molecules within the front surface to depths of several microns. They become an integral part of the lens and not a coating that can wear or rub off. The process of imbibing can be illustrated by imaging a piece of standard laboratory filter paper saturated with the photochromic compounds and then allowed to air dry. The result is a paper with a compound evenly dispersed throughout. By placing the paper on the lens surface and heating both lens and paper, the compound will transfer and imbibe into the lens surface. Penetration depth of the compound is in the region of 100-150 microns. The advantage of the system is that no matter what the prescription is, the tint density is uniform. Unlike glass photochromic, resin photochromic lenses, begin activation instantly as they are exposed to sunlight with no break-in period. Over a period of approximately 2 years resin photochromic will degrade due to their exposure to UV radiation, unlike glass where the reaction is locked in permanently, for the life of the lens.

DISPENSING TIPS FOR PHOTOCHROMATIC LENSES

Photochromic lenses are not as effective in hot climate. When temperature increases, the reaction slows. So they are not recommended to replace sunglasses. However, they are useful lens to have, as the variation allows comfortable vision in almost all conditions with one pair of glasses.

Photochromic lenses do not lighten instantaneously when going from a bright to a dim area. For this reason, the elderly often experience problems wearing photochromic as the need for good illumination increases with age. The convenience gained from a darkened lens in a bright environment is offset by the inconvenience experienced when coming into a darker indoor from outside.

Also because the photochromic do not always return to their maximum transmission, the additional reduction in illumination when driving at night may prove hazardous.

No coating that absorbs UV light should ever be used on the front surface of a photochromic lens. Such a coating interferes with the darkening of the lens. Such a coating can, however, be placed on the rear surface without interference.

Anti-reflection coating will not reduce the range of the photochromic cycles but as with any lens, will increase the transmission in both the lightened and darkened status. Theoretically, a multicoated photochromic lens will transmit as much light as an uncoated clear glass lens, in its lightening state.

Photochromic lenses may be treated either through chemtempering for optimum mechanical strength, or air tempering. In the latter case, the treated lenses become lighter a little more slowly and darken rather more in the sun.

When replacing a single lens, the problem of a color mismatch between the lenses often arises. There are three useful points to remember in order to avoid this problem:

1. Always make sure that the new lens is of the same type as the old one, i.e., same brand, same thickness etc.
2. If the old lens has been chemtempered, have it re-strengthened along with as the new lens.
3. If the old lens has not been treated in anyway, place it with the new lens in boiling water for half an hour (The infrared in the hot water restores original clearness to the old lens).

POLAROID LENSES

Under normal lighting conditions, light waves vibrate and travel in all directions —horizontally, vertically and also everywhere in between. When incident light either from direct sunlight or artificial light hit non-metallic surface such as sheet of glass, surface of still water or wet roads at a given angle, they become partially polarized, their vibration being restricted to two mutually perpendicular directions only. If the surface is horizontal, the direction of vibration will also be horizontal and intensifying the effect of polarized light on the eyes. Polarized lenses block those horizontally reflected light which causes glare, while allowing vertically aligned light to transmit **(Fig. 7.8)**. The principle of polarized lens is best illustrated by observing venetian blinds which blocks light at certain angles, while allows light to transmit through it at certain other angle as shown in **Figure 7.9**.

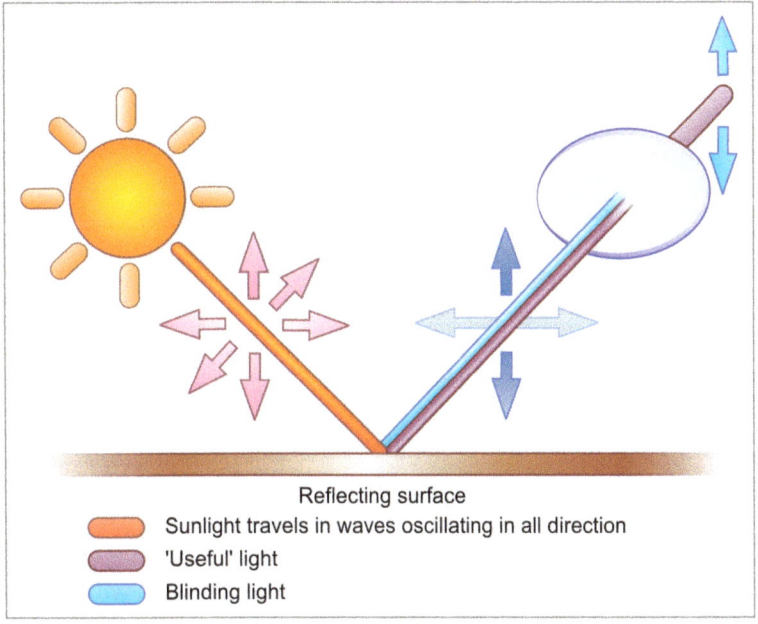

Fig. 7.8: Polaroid lens allows only useful vertical light waves

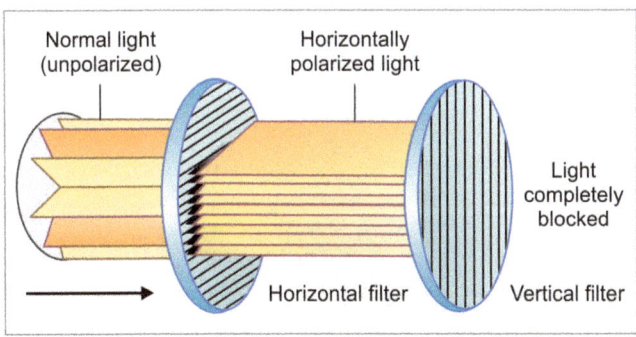

Fig. 7.9: Polarized lens works like venetian blinds

APPLICATION OF POLARIZED LENSES

Polarizing filters are created by stretching sheets of polyvinyl alcohol (PVA) so that its molecules align in long directional chains. The PVA is then passed through an iodine solution where the light absorbing iodine molecules attach to the molecular chains forming the microscopic blinds. The film so prepared is sandwiched in the lens **(Fig. 7.10)**. The back surface of the lens is cast first and the precurved Polaroid film is placed on the cast part and then liquid material is injected over. Polarizing filters are aligned 90° to the angle of the polarized light.

As spectacle lenses are designed to eliminate the polarized light in the horizontal plane, the filter is placed vertically in the eyewear or eye rim. This means that the filter must be properly aligned during surfacing and edging layout, otherwise filters will not work properly.

ADVANTAGES OF POLAROID LENSES

1. Filters glares
2. Enhances contrast and depth perception
3. Reduces eye strain, greater comfort
4. Improves visual acuity, provides safety
5. Eyes feel rested
6. Realistic visual perception **(Fig. 7.11)**
7. Reduces reflection
8. Comfortable and attractive – looking sun wear.

TINTS VS. POLARIZED LENSES

Although, darkly tinted sunglasses may reduce brightness, they do not remove glares like polarized lenses. In addition, dark sunglasses without added ultraviolet protection may cause more damage to the patients eyes than not wearing sunglasses at all. The darkness of the lens can cause the pupil to dilate,

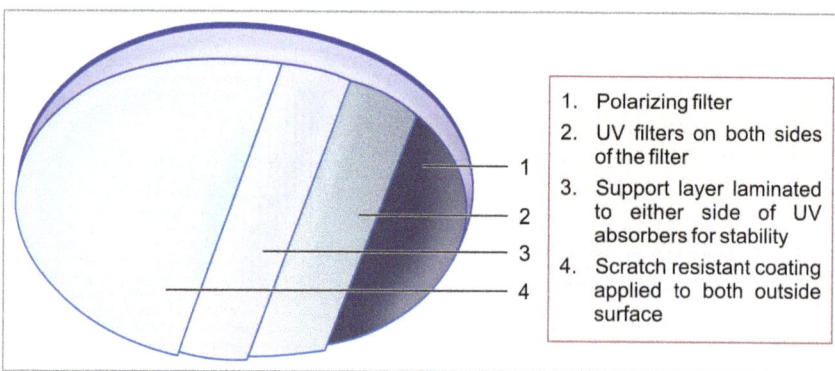

Fig. 7.10: Composing of polaroid lens

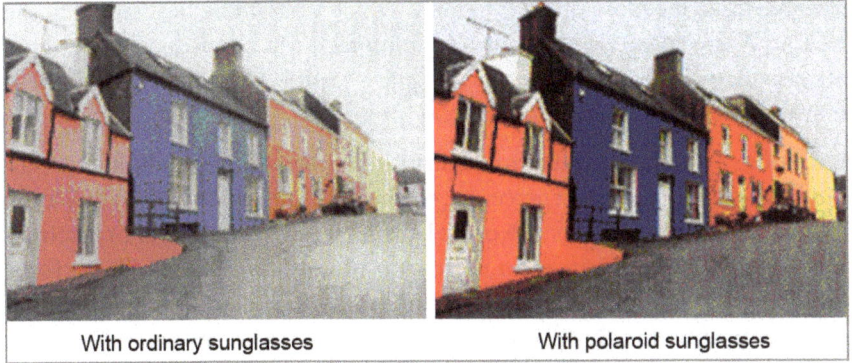

Fig. 7.11: Realistic color perception

letting more ultraviolet rays into the inner parts of the eyes. Polarized lenses solve both problems by eliminating glares and filtering out harmful ultraviolet light because the filter reduces the polarized glare and also has UV absorbing properties.

DISPENSING TIPS FOR POLAROID LENSES

In order for polarizing filter to work effectively, the polarizing filter is placed in the path of reflected lights with its transmission axis at right angles to the reflecting surface at vertical. It absorbs reflected light which are parallel to horizontal surface. The straight forward meaning is that the filter must be positioned correctly during surfacing and edging layout to work effectively. To facilitate correct positioning of the polarizing filter, the manufacturer marks the direction of the transmission axis on the uncut or semi-finished blank so that it can be accurately positioned during the manufacturing and assembling process. Some manufacturer prefers to indicate the correct orientation of the lens by marking horizontal meridian. It is, therefore, important to know which meridian is marked before lens setting is processed.

In case of multifocal or progressive lenses the transmission axis of the polarizing film is oriented in the vertical meridian with respect to the segment setting or the meridian line of the progressive surface.

However, polarized lenses may react adversely with liquid crystal display (LCDs) found on the dashboard of some cars or in other places such as digital screen on automatic letter machines. The problem with LCDs is that when viewed through polarized lenses from a certain angle, they can be invisible.

PRESCRIBING TINTS

The scope and application of color lenses are huge and varied. With usage ranging from pure aesthetics, fashion and sports to medical and safety applications, and with the infinite variety of fixed tints, graduated tints and variable tints, it can be difficult to know which tint can be best suited to the wearer. While cosmetic choice is a primary factor in choosing a color, there are also many other reasons for the opticians to prescribe tinted lenses. These may include the followings:

Luminous transmission factor: Transmission level is specified in terms of luminous transmission as a percentage of the light transmitted. For example, LT 80 brown tint lens transmits 80% of the light averaged over the visible spectrum. The color of a tinted lens is an indication of its absorption characteristics but the exact transmission can only be found by measuring on a scanning spectrophotometer. By specifying the light transmission factor precisely, corrections can be made easily if the tint is too light or too dark.

Light sensitivity: Light sensitivity or photophobia is a common eye complaint. It can result from several different conditions. Many a times a patient will complain of light sensitivity, for which no logical explanation can be given. Most of these individual tends to be fair skinned, with blue eyes. The treatment is the judicious use of tinted glasses to relieve their symptoms. Usually those with some light sensitivity will choose grey, green and blue and reject orange and yellow. The reason is likely to be that yellow and orange are at or near the peak spectral sensitivity of the eye. On the scale of light sensitivity, even green can be too bright for some people.

Contrast enhancement: Contrast filters are generally red, orange, yellow and light green. They tend to allow the transmission of light that is the same as the color of the filter and promote tonal separation in that color. At the same time they tend to suppress other color. The bright contrasting effect is achieved by absorbing blue and UV—both of which contribute to a veiling background haze. Contrast enhancement can be achieved with green, yellow, brown and red tinted lenses – the choice again depends on color preference and use. Yellow has a limited application in bright sunlight because it transmits visible light at the eyes peak sensitivity.

Reduced migraines: Patient who experiences migraines may be hypersensitive to the visual stimuli. Color filters can reduce symptoms caused by these stimuli. The choice of lens color may also be an important factor to reduce migraines. In one study, children who wore lenses with either pink or a blue tint experience migraines less frequently after 1 month. At 4 months, however children wearing only pink tinted lens continued to experience migraines less frequently.

Reading comfort and performance: Tinted lenses may filter out certain light frequencies and reduce the amount of information the eyes absorb. Some researchers believe that by reducing the amount of information, the brain can process better what the eyes see. Another study of children and adults with learning disabilities showed that the rate of reading was significantly faster in the subjects who read with glasses that had a colored overlay compared with those who read with glasses without a color overlay. Research by Optometrist Mr. Harold A. Solan from New York, has demonstrated that blue light filters are superior to the other color filters for this purpose. It caused improvement in the number of fixations and regression and rate of reading in children with learning disabilities.

Driving factors: Lenses for driving must not be too dark, as they reduce visual acuity. It is essential to offer protection to the eyes while driving in order to see better, react quickly to dangerous conditions and improve safety. A brown tinted lens is ideal for drivers for day time driving as they reduce the transmission of blue light. But it is too dark to use in the night. Night driving lenses would typically have a yellow tint or amber tint with antireflection coating which may improve contrast and reduce glare.

There may be a possibility that the subject may not be very comfortable with any tint and he rejects all the colors. But the normal requirements of protections still apply—everyone should protect their eyes in bright sunlight. In practice, a neutral density grey filter would be used by this group. Contrarily, if all the colors are equally liked, then the tint can be chosen on optical principles, say when required for sunglass, a brown tint which has UV absorption and contrast enhancing properties would be better.

BLUE LIGHT AND BLUE CUT LENSES

The term "blue light" is the simplification of blue, indigo and violet light. They lie at the shorter wavelength of visible spectrum between 380 nm to 500 nm and are the neighbor of UV light. Blue light reaches the eyes in totality and carries huge amount of energy with it, so they are said to have significant damaging effect on eye. While natural exposure to blue light during the day boosts people's energy, alertness and mood, elongated exposure to blue light transmitted through screen devices during evening or night time can disrupt circadian rhythm and cause various health issues including sleep disorder. Chronic exposure to blue light may risk early age related macular degeneration (ARMD) and other pathologies. However, not all blue light is bad. The spectrum of blue light lies between 380 nm to 500 nm is divided into two classes as shown in **Figure 7.12**.
- Low energy visible blue (LEV blue)
- High energy visible blue (HEV blue)

The division is around 435 nm—all blue light below 435 nm falls under HEV blue light and all blue light above 435 nm falls under LEV blue light. LEV blue lies above 435 nm and gives the perception of blue–turquoise light. We need LEV blue for our well-being. HEV blue lies below 435 nm and gives the perception of blue-violet light. We need to prevent HEV blue for our well-being.

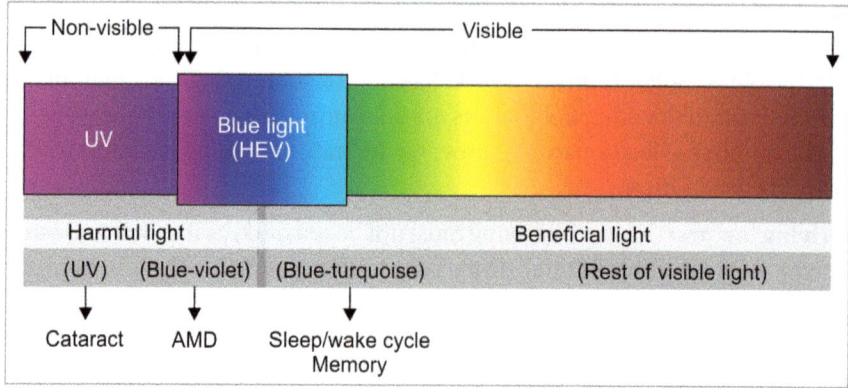

Fig. 7.12: Spectrum of blue light

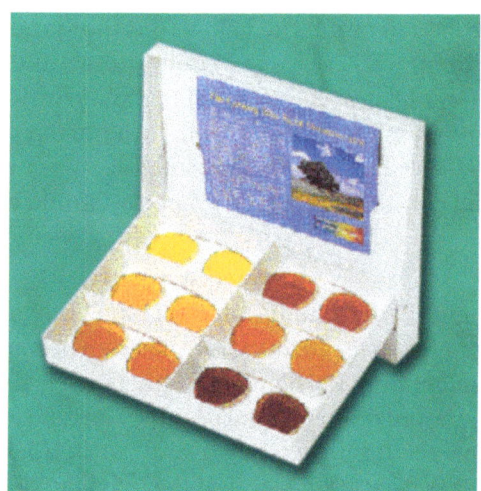

Fig. 7.13: Corning CPF lenses

The harmfulness of HEV blue light can be minimized by the use of selective or protective filtering lenses and also be altering the properties of lens material that absorbs UV and HEV Blue light and allow the transmission of LEV blue with other visible lights. Additionally, it can also work to increase contrast and thereby improves vision quality. Similar effect can also be achieved by applying blue cut anti-reflection coating on the lens surface. Corning has introduced a range of CPF photochromatic filters **(Fig 7.13)** which includes CPF 450, CPF 511, CPF 527 and CPF 550 which have been successfully prescribed to protect the eyes from blue light in cataract, diabetic retinopathy, macular degeneration, retinitis pigmentosa, corneal dystrophy, albinism, aniridia or glaucoma.

Sunlight is the main source of blue light, but there are also many man-made, indoor sources of blue light, including fluorescent and LED lighting and flat-screen televisions and many digital gadgets used in daily life.

☞ Multiple Choice Questions (MCQs)

1. The visible spectrum in the electromagnetic spectrum ranges from …..
   a. 380 nm to 780 nm
   b. 280 nm to 760 nm
   c. 420 nm to 880 nm
   d. 300 nm to 700 nm

2. The portion of electromagnetic spectrum that is of ophthalmic concern are……
   a. Ultraviolet rays
   b. Visible rays
   c. Infrared rays
   d. All of the above

3. Which of the following wavelength of UV rays is the cause of the most concern for ophthalmic professional?
   a. UV – A
   b. UV – B
   c. UV – C
   d. All of the above

4. When the light is incident on the lens surface, what happens to the light?
   a. Light is refracted
   b. Light is reflected
   c. Light is absorbed
   d. All of the above

5. The percentage of light transmitted through an uncoated crown glass lenses is…
   a. 99%
   b. 98.2%
   c. 91.2%
   d. 96%

6. Which of the following is the neutral density filter?
   a. Red
   b. Grey
   c. Blue
   d. Green

7. Which of the tint is most commonly prescribed in neurological problems?
   a. Brown
   b. Yellow
   c. Blue
   d. Pink

8. Which of the following tint is often prescribed to enhance the contrast visual acuity?
   a. Orange
   b. Blue
   c. Grey
   d. Violet

Answers							
1. a	2. d	3. a	4. d	5. c	6. b	7. d	8. a

Chapter 8

Anti-reflection Coated Lens

The normal eye is easily adapted to different lighting conditions. Thus, the loss of light due to reflection is usually not serious enough to reduce visibility except where poor lighting condition already exist. It is the reflected light which enters the pupil of the eye along the same path as the light used in "seeing" an object that is of primary importance. Whenever light is incident on the boundary between two medium, some light is reflected and some is transmitted, and the transmitted light undergoes refraction into the second medium. Anti-reflection coating are applied on the lens surface to efficiently manipulate the light transmission and reflection through it. It has been seen that the surface reflectance can be reduced by coating the lens with a film of some materials having a lower refractive index than that of the lens. Although, there are now two reflections—one at the exposed surface of the film and another at the lens surface, their combined effect produces less reflection than the uncoated surface. The result is, patient experiences a marked sensation of improved vision. There is no doubt that anti-reflection coating leads to greater patient comfort.

■ THE REFLECTION OF LIGHT

Dr Rayton presented some of the problems encountered due to reflections of light in spectacle lenses. There are four definable sources of reflection that can cause annoyance to the spectacle lens wearer:

1. **Frontal reflection:** Frontal reflection occurs when some of the light incident on the front surface is reflected back towards an observer as shown in **Figure 8.1B**. This can be disconcerting for the observer, as the wearer's eyes are difficult to observe. Communications between human relies just not on spoken or written words but also by facial expressions, much of which are centered on the eye's reactions. Inability to see the eyes of a person you are talking to can be rather "off-putting" as one cannot deduce whether what is being said is actually being understood. These reflections are also annoying from purely a cosmetic point of view as they detract from the overall appearance.
2. **Backward reflection:** Backward reflections occur when some of the light behind the patient is reflected from the back surface of the lens into his eyes as shown in **Figure 8.1A**. This can be annoying at times when reduced lighting conditions are encountered such as at dusk or while driving at night.

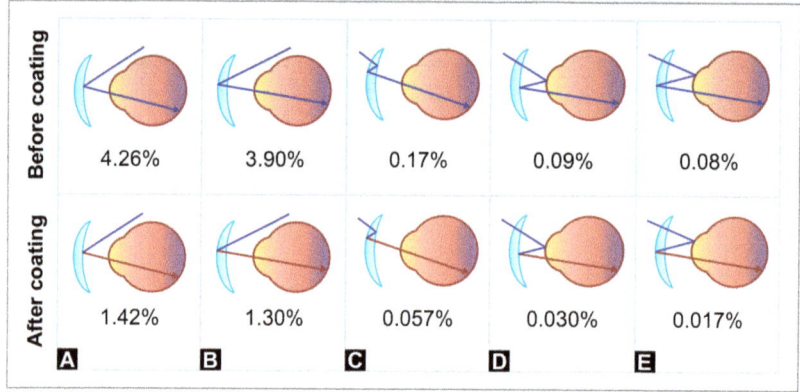

Fig. 8.1: Reflection of light
  A. Light reflected from the rear lens surface into the eye
  B. Light reflected from the front lens surface into the eye
  C. Light entering the eye after double reflection within lens
  D. Light reflected by cornea to rear lens surface and back into the eye
  E. Light reflected by cornea to front lens surface and back into the eye

3. **Internal reflection:** Internal reflection is caused by light being reflected between the two lens surfaces as shown in **Figure 8.1C**. The amount of reflection caused in this manner depends upon the power and position of the lens in front of the eyes.
4. **Corneal reflection:** Corneal reflection is caused by light being reflected from the corneal surface and then interacting with the lens surfaces as shown in **Figures 8.1D and E**.

While frontal reflections would appear only to be a cosmetic problem they do reduce the amount of light transmitted through to the eyes. Backward, internal and corneal reflections all cause ghost imaging that in turn can lead to reduce visual acuity due to blurring and reduced contrast, which overall reduces the effectiveness of the prescription lens and thereby reduces its efficiency.

PRINCIPLE OF ANTI-REFLECTION COATING

Anti-reflection coating is applied on the lens surface to reduce the loss of light due to reflection and increase the light transmittance through the lens to the eyes. To understand how it is achieved, we need to remember "Quantum theory" that tells that the light travels in waves **(Fig. 8.2)** similar to those in the ocean.

The "Principle of Optical Interference" explains that there are two types of optical interference:
- Destructive Interference, and
- Constructive Interference.

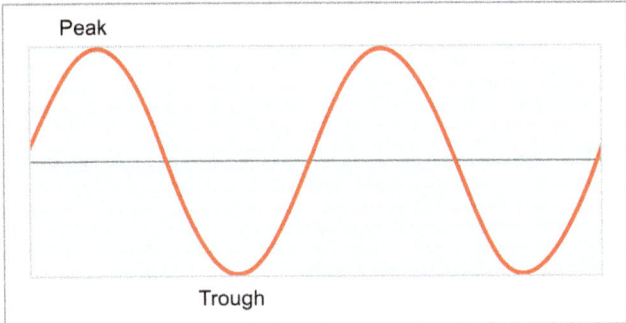

Fig. 8.2: Light wave

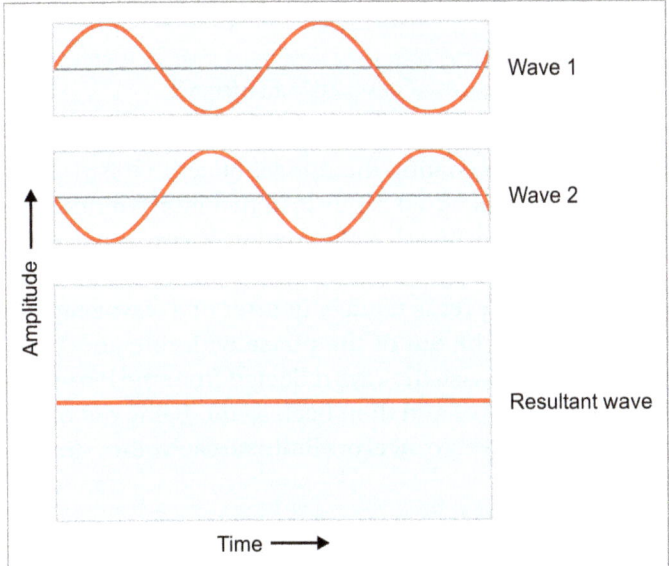

Fig. 8.3: Destructive interference

Destructive interference occurs when the light waves are traveling out of phase with each other. When this occurs the peak of the wave is lined up with the trough of another wave and they virtually cancel each other out as shown in **Figure 8.3**.

With constructive interference we have the opposite effect happening. In this case the light waves are traveling in phase with each other so that the peaks and troughs of one wave line up with the peaks and troughs of another wave. They are now working together creating one larger wave as shown in **Figure 8.4**.

In a two layer coating, the outer layer is made of a low refractive index and the inner layer is made of a high refractive index material compared to the substrate.

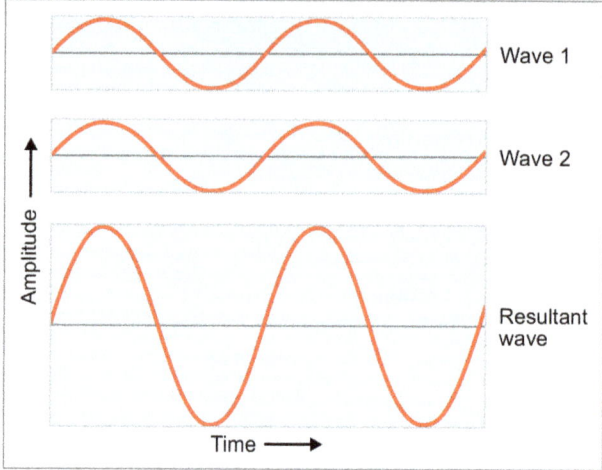

Fig. 8.4: Constructive interference

With anti-reflection coating the optical effect that is used to reduce the surface reflection is based on destructive interference. It works by interposing a transparent layer, i.e. the coating; we cause two reflections—the first from the surface layer itself and the second from the lens surface. If the thickness of the layer is made a quarter of a wavelength thick, the two reflected rays will be out of the phase with one another by half a wavelength. This is because the rays reflected from the lens surface have to travel through the layer and then back again. Being out of phase with one another they effectively cancel or eliminate each other, thus destroying the reflection.

■ SINGLE LAYER ANTI-REFLECTION COATING

The simple principle of single layer anti-reflection coating is that the substrate (lens) is coated with a thin layer of material so that reflection from the outer surface of the film and the outer surface of the substrate cancel each other by destructive interference. To achieve this we take the advantage of the undulatory nature of light by creating opposition of phases between reflected waves **(Fig. 8.5)**.

If we place a thin coating on the lens, the light beam, which is a series of waves, hits the coating and breaks up into reflected waves and refracted waves. The refracted waves then hit the lens and split second time into reflected and refracted waves. By a careful calculation of the thickness and index, in such a way that the first series of reflected waves and the second are super imposed while being out of the phase by half a wavelength, we obtain mutual cancellation. Light which is not reflected is refracted.

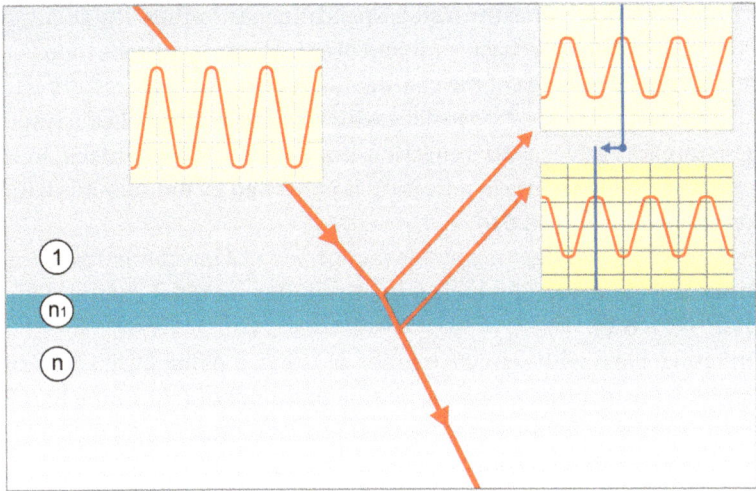

Fig. 8.5: Principle of anti-reflection coating

However, in practice it is impossible to attain total extinction of reflection just by depositing a single layer of coating on the lens. In fact, the reflection could be almost eliminated by meeting two conditions:

1. The refractive index of the coating is the square root of that of the lens material.
$$^n film = \sqrt{^n Substrate}$$

2. The thickness of the coating, multiplied by its refractive index, is exactly one-quarter of a wavelength of light or any odd number of quarter wavelengths.

Unfortunately, this is not always obtainable. Crown glass with a refractive index of 1.523 would need a material with an index of 1.234, whereas the most suitable material available for glass is Magnesium Fluoride which has a refractive index of around 1.38. So it is not very well suited for crown glasses but its performance is better on higher index materials. Also the two necessary conditions can be met for only one wavelength. This is the reason why single layer anti-reflection coating cannot reduce the reflectance in the entire range of visible spectrum. Single layer coatings are designed to give their maximum effect in the middle and brightest region of the visible spectrum. The reflectance gradually increases towards both violet and red ends of the spectrum. As a result, the coated surface presents the characteristics of purplish appearance which is described as bloom.

▬ MULTILAYER ANTI-REFLECTION COATING

The limitations of the single layer antireflection coating can be overcome by multilayer coating which are now capable of almost extinguishing surface reflections from one end of the visible spectrum to the other. The coating may be two layers or more. The basic problem of a single layer antireflection coating is that the refractive index of the coating material is too high, resulting in too strong reflection from the first surface which cannot be cancelled completely by the comparatively weaker reflection from the substrate surface. In a two layer coating, the first surface reflection is cancelled by interference with two weaker reflections **(Fig. 8.6)**.

In a two layer coating, the outer layer is made of a low refractive index and the inner layer is made of a high refractive index material compared to the substrate **(Fig. 8.7)**.

On crown glass with refractive index of 1.523, the first layer of coating is applied with the material which has a refractive index of 1.70. Either beryllium oxide or magnesium oxide is used for this layer. And the top layer is coated with magnesium fluoride which has a refractive index of 1.38. Both beryllium oxide and magnesium oxide are soft materials and will not produce very durable coating. Although, it allows some freedom in the choice of coating materials and can give very low reflectance, the two layer coating is very restrictive in its design. As a consequence multi-layer antireflection coatings have been developed to allow the refractive index of each layer to be chosen. The complex computer design techniques were developed to make multilayer coating based on the simple principles of interference and phase shifts. All methods consider the combined effect of various film elements. Each layer is influenced by the optical properties of the layer next to it. The properties of that layer are influenced by its environment. Clearly this represents at least a complex series of matrix

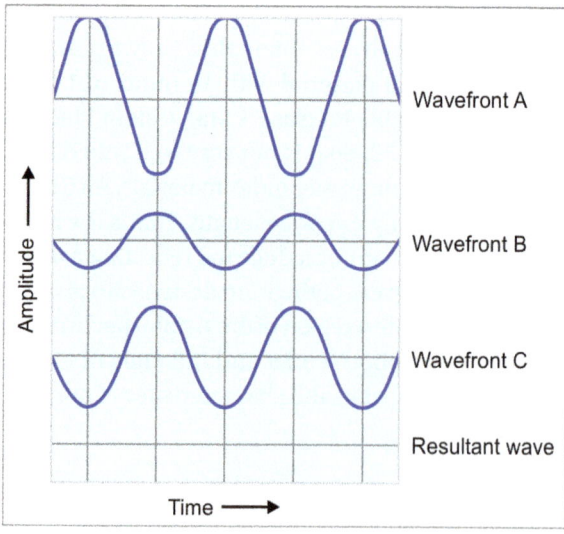

Fig. 8.6: Interference in two layer coating

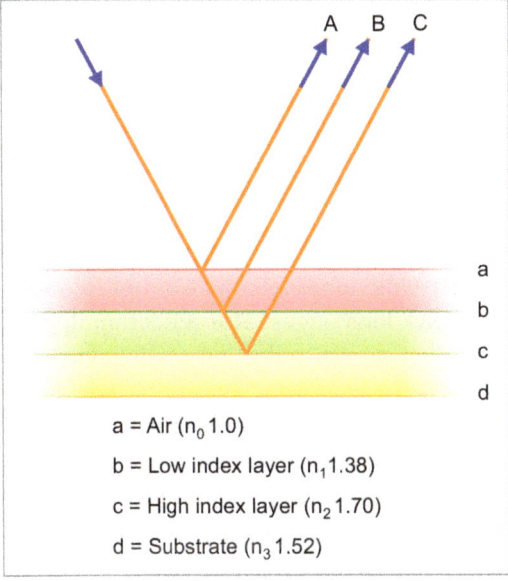

Fig. 8.7: Two layer coating

multiplication where each matrix corresponds to a single layer. The efficiency is not necessarily directly related to the number of layers used, rather on correct selection of coating materials for refractive index, the thickness with which the layers are applied, and the adherence to the previous layer of the materials are all qualifications for an efficient multiple coating.

ADVANTAGES OF ANTI-REFLECTION COATING

Primarily reasons for recommending anti-reflection coating to the eyewear consumer are:

1. People see better with anti-reflection coated lenses as anti-reflection coated lenses transmit more lights. Conventional glass or plastic gains 8% in light transmission. High index lenses gain even more 11% to 16% depending on the materials. Increased light means wearer sees things brighter and clearer, with crisper details.
2. While looking at a person wearing uncoated lenses, we see reflection of light that is actually coming from the front surface of the lenses. This can be disconcerting for the observer, as the wearer's eyes are difficult to observe, creating a barrier between the observer and the wearer. By getting rid of the reflections, the lenses seem to "disappear" into the frame.
3. Ghost images are a common experience with uncoated lenses, particularly while driving at night. These visual annoyances appear as dull images created by reflections coming from the internal lens surfaces. With minus correction, ghost images are crisp and reflected on the side of the light image towards

the optical centre. With plus lenses, ghost images are larger, less distinct and appear away from the optical centre. Most patients drive vehicles and understand the advantage of anti-reflection coating eliminating ghost images.
4. Reflections from back lens surfaces can also be annoying. This is most noticeable with sun lenses because the dark lens acts like a mirror. Backside reflections are also more prominent with aspheric lenses as their flatter inside surface reflects more light.
5. Strong minus lenses can produce a "Coke bottle" look caused by light reflecting from thick lens edges. The reflection appears as a series of concentric rings. Modern anti-reflection coatings virtually eliminate these unsightly rings.
6. Anti-reflection coating has become popular in recent years. As a result, there is a growing perception among consumers that, quality eyewear include anti-reflection coating. Offices that do not routinely recommend anti-reflection coated lenses, risk having patient learn about it from a friend, neighbour or a competitors advertising.

ANTI-REFLECTION COATING OF PRETINTED LENSES

Glass lenses in which the tint is in the lens material itself, may also be anti-reflection coated. This is quite advantageous in several situations:
1. If a person desires a light tint in his lenses and yet it is felt that night vision is hindered by it, anti-reflection coating may return the glass to its previous non-tinted transmission. For example, pink tint may reduce the lens transmission from 92% to 88%. Anti-reflection coating on the lens will bring the transmission back to at least 92%, while multi-layer coating may increase the transmission to above 92%. In spite of the increased transmission, the pink lens maintains its characteristic of light coloured appearance.
2. Sun lenses may be antireflection coated to advantage as well. For example, the patient may find reflections from the back surface of the sun lens disturbing. This is a genuine complaint because of the reflection coming from behind. An anti-reflection coating allows majority of light coming from behind the wearer to pass on through the lens without being reflected back into the eyes.
3. Photochromatic lenses may be anti-reflection coated. This will increase both maximum and minimum transmission by a certain amount. The lens will transmit more light in both the lightened and the darkened state. It also helps when lenses are dark by reducing backside reflections from dark lenses.

DISPENSING TIPS

In dispensing anti-reflection coated lenses, always remember not to sell half pair lens. Whenever only one lens is required, most laboratories will strip anti-reflection coating from the old lens and recoat both lenses together for an exact colour match. Never use a stock anti-reflection coated lens for one eye and order custom anti-reflection coating for the other. Inevitably, there will be a slight colour difference in the anti-reflection coating. The difference in colour has no effect on vision but is always noticed by the patient.

Be sure to explain that anti-reflection lenses must never be cleaned dry, as this can scratch the coating. The best cleaner is one that is made especially for anti-reflection coated lenses. Patient should not use acetone, windex, caustic solution or soaps to clean the anti-reflection coated lenses. Make sure that every eyewear patient going through the office gets an explanation and demonstration of anti-reflection coatings benefits. This ensures that every patient understands you are trained and skilled in dispensing what has become accepted as the most advanced modern eye wear available.

TECHNOLOGY FOR APPLYING ANTI-REFLECTION COATING

Anti-reflection coating is applied to the lens surface to reduce the surface reflection of light. The reflectance of the surface decreases as the difference between the refractive indices of the media which is on either side of the surface decreases. This is achieved by creating the stack of the material on both the surface of the lens having low refractive index. Applying anti-reflection coating requires great technical expertise and very high quality pure coating material. The lens to be coated must be absolutely free of surface defects, perfectly cleaned and rid of dust or any other impurities before they are placed for anti-reflection coating. All lenses are cleaned manually and ultrasonically in an air conditioned, pressurized, dust free room. Resin lenses are treated with hard coating before putting for coating.

Mainly there are three different processes that are commonly applied for anti-reflection coating:
1. Vacuum coating
2. Sputter coating
3. Sol-gel coating

After the pre-coating processes, the lenses are placed in the lens holder. The lens holder is placed inside the vacuum chamber where crucibles of coating material are heated until it is melt and then further heated to evaporate. The material evaporates and travels through the vacuum to deposit on the lens surface. The crucibles lie at the center of the curvature of domed lens holder to ensure that the film thickness is build up at the same rate upon each lens surface. When one surface is coated, the lenses must be reversed in order to coat the other surface.

The different coating materials like silicon oxides, titanium, zirconium and magnesium fluoride are held in sealed crucibles within the box chamber which are opened in sequence automatically.

Once the anti-reflective stack is applied; an anti-static and hydrophobic or hydrophilic layer can also be applied on top.

Temperature control is very critical for the adhesion of coating with substrate. Extremely low pressure is created inside the chamber by removing the air from it and a very high temperature is being ensured. Mineral glass lenses can be heated up to 300 °C (570 °F), but plastics heated above 100 °C (210 °F). With glass material it is possible that the coating can be baked after deposition to make them strongly adhered.

Anti-reflective coating can also be applied by Sputter coating and Sol-gel process. Sputter coating process is more suited for lower volume of lenses. The coating material is placed inside the sputter in the form of block of metal and a gas is injected into the chamber and is excited. The excited gas molecules hit the block of metal with high energy that allows the metal material dispersed onto the lens surface to produce the coating of alternative high and low index film. Sol-gel process involves applying anti reflection coating using dipping method. After dipping the films are heated and allowed to absorb water vapor so that reaction takes place that liberates the solvent. The lenses with their coating in gel form are next tempered in a furnace at very high temperature. Residual water is driven off and a hard film of metal oxide is formed from the gel.

Multiple Choice Questions (MCQs)

1. **When should lenses be tinted if they are to be coated with anti-reflective coating?**
   a. After the coating is applied
   b. Before the coating is applied
   c. It does not matter whether it is before or after the coating is applied
   d. Lenses to be coated with anti-reflective coating should never be tinted

2. **The primary reason for applying anti-reflective coating is...**
   a. To manipulate the light transmission and reflection through the lens
   b. To minimize the refraction of light through the lens
   c. To cancel the effect of out of phase waves of light
   d. None of the above

3. **Which of the following type of light reflection usually does not cause ghost image?**
   a. Reflection caused by back surface of the lens
   b. Reflection caused by corneal surface and then interacting with the lens surface
   c. Reflection caused by front surface of the lens
   d. Internal reflection caused by light being reflected between two lens surfaces

4. Which of the following laws is the basic principle behind anti-reflection coating?
   a. The law of Constructive Interference
   b. The law of Destructive Interference
   c. The law of Reflection
   d. Fermat's Principle

5. Which of the following technology is commonly used for mass production of anti-reflection coated spectacle lenses?
   a. Vacuum Coating
   b. Sputter Coating
   c. Sol-gel Coating
   d. All of the above

Answers

| 1. b | 2. a | 3. c | 4. b | 5. a |

Chapter 9

Aspheric Lenses

The term 'aspheric' has been widely used in recent years to describe the surfaces of the various lens designs. The literal meaning of the term 'aspheric' means 'not spheric', which means cylinder surfaces or toroidal surfaces used for astigmatic correction are also a type of aspheric surface. Often 'progressive addition lens' surface is also described as aspheric. In terms of lens designing the term 'aspheric' is reserved for the surfaces that are rotationally symmetrical, but at the same time not spherical, generated by the revolution of symmetrical, but non-circular curves about its axis of symmetry. A change in curvature is noticed across the lens surface, rather than constant curvature like a spherical surface. The change is the same in all direction or meridians of the lens. The surface is spherical at the center of the lens but as you move away from the center into the paraxial and peripheral zone, it turns into the aspheric surface progressively depending upon the degree of asphericity. The asphericity in plus lens is achieved by flattening the front surface of the lens or by steepening the back surface of the lens. In case of minus power asphericity is achieved by steepening front surface of the lens away from the center or flattening the back surface of the lens away from the center. Using the "asphericity" the lens designers are able to produce flatter lens and thinner lenses that also provide improved peripheral vision.

- The off-axis performance of lens improves considerably.
- The lens looks flatter which makes the eyes look more natural due to reduced magnifications or minifications.
- Flatter lens fits better into the frame, making the spectacle look more appealing as shown in **Figure 9.1**, thereby offering the wearer a wider choice of frames to choose from.

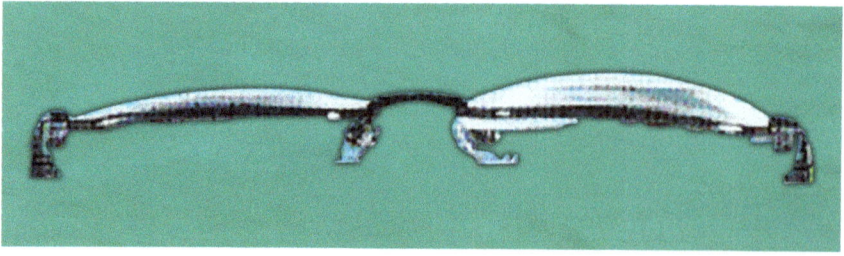

Fig. 9.1: Comparison between aspheric and spheric surface

- If the aspheric lenses are coupled with high index lens material, it will definitely provide thinner, lighter and flatter lenses that look cosmetically the best.

The degree of asphericity is defined by eccentricity or E-value. Eccentricity is the number derived from the ratio of the length of the short axis to the length of the long axis of an object that defines the shape of the asphericity **(Fig. 9.2)**.

Higher the number, higher is the degree of asphericity. The **Table 9.1** shows the E-value of various shapes.

It is possible that higher degree of asphericity may create more surface astigmatism and degrade the lens performance rather than improving it for a given lens prescription. It implies that there must be some reference to select the appropriate degree of asphericity. One of the justifiable approaches that can be thought over is the shape of the corneal. The average eccentricity value of human cornea is between 0.4 to 0.6. If we can mimic a lens surface with that of corneal surface, probably we get a most appropriate answer. But this may not be applied in all cases of abnormal corneas or abnormally higher lens prescription for various reasons.

Another approach can be developed based upon the focal power of the lens. Higher focal power of lens will fetch higher e-value aspheric lens design and lower focal power of the lens will fetch lower e-value aspheric lens design. The problem in this case is no lens manufacture provides precise information regarding their lens design. Moreover, it also means that a set of lens power will be grouped together for a given e-value. Within a group only a limited number

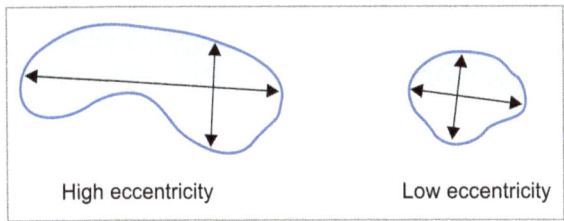

Fig. 9.2: Higher eccentricity vs lower eccentricity

Table 9.1: E-value of various shapes

Shape	E-value
Sphere	0
Ellipsoid	0.1–0.9
Paraboloid	1
Hyperboloid	> 1
Average cornea	0.4–0.6

of lens powers that are located near the center of the power range associated with each e-value will deliver the desired performance.

It leaves us with no other option than to customize the degree of asphericity for a given lens prescription. The lens designer selects the required base curve needed to generate the desired flatness, calculates the power error and astigmatic error across the entire lens surface that will result because of the selected base curve using computer software and generate the desired asphericity to compensate for the same. The lens so made will not only provide flatter lens that will look good cosmetically but will also be provide good optics.

However, before taking the decision on appropriate degree of asphericity, the designer must make necessary compensation for lens size as larger size lens would need higher e-value lens than the smaller size.

■ WHY ASPHERIC?

Several lens aberrations influence the quality of peripheral vision through a spectacle lens. The most important among them is the oblique astigmatism which is of great concern for the lens designer. It happens when the rays of light strike the paraxial and peripheral portion of the lens obliquely, resulting in two focal lines from each single object point. The dioptric difference between these two focal lines is known as the astigmatic error of the lens. The effect of this aberration is the reduction in wearer's field of clearer vision through the lens. In conventional spherical lenses, the choice of base curve is the only way to minimize the effect of oblique astigmatism. But when the flatter curve is selected with an objective to make the lens flatter, it introduces significant amount of aberration and deteriorates the peripheral vision quality further as shown in **Figure 9.3**. The lens designer applies appropriate degree of asphericity to minimize the effect of aberration and thus improves the quality of vision.

■ ASPHERIC LENS DESIGN

A spherical surface has the same curvature in any direction across the entire surface, whereas aspheric surface becomes progressively flatter or, steeper away from the center of the lens, i.e., the tangential meridian of the lens. Aspheric surface changes very little around the circumference of the lens, which is the sagittal plane of the lens perpendicular to the tangential plane **(Fig. 9.4)**. This difference in surface curvature produces surface astigmatism, the effect of which increases as the eyes move away from the center of the lens. The aspheric surface literally produces cylinder power away from its center which counteracts and neutralizes the oblique astigmatism produced by looking through the off-axis portion of the lens. The degree of asphericity also increases as you go more away from the center of the lens to minimize the effect of increasing oblique astigmatism.

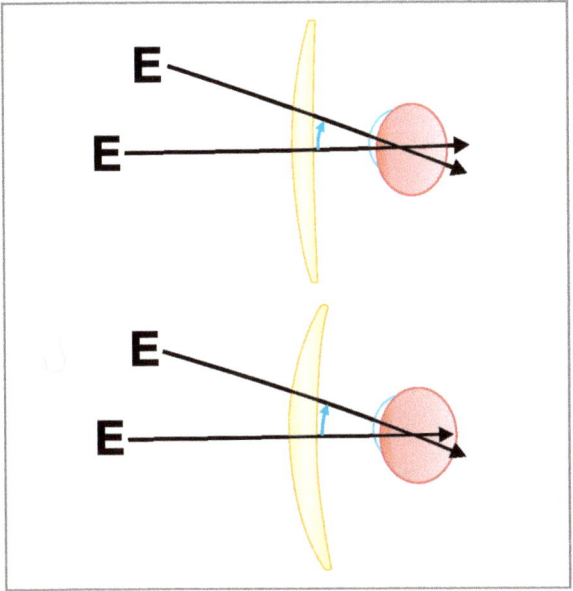

Fig. 9.3: The steeper lens provides better off-axis optics, while the flatter lens provides better cosmetics

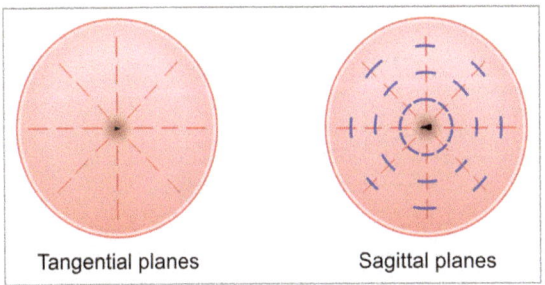

Fig. 9.4: Tangential and sagittal planes of refraction

Three-dimensional aspheric curves are produced by rotating a non-circular curve about an axis of symmetry of conicoid solid to generate conic sections that include the parabola, hyperbola, and the ellipse **(Fig. 9.5)**. Since axis of symmetry divides the cone into two equal halves, all aspheric surfaces are "rotationally-symmetrical." All these sections of cone generate the aspheric curves of different eccentricities with near spherical central region, the front curve value of which is utilized for lens power and surfacing calculations. More sophisticated aspheric surfaces can be generated using mathematical formulas described by polynomial equations. The surface generated out of the mathematical formulas offers more flexibility to the lens designer than a simple conicoid surface. **Figure 9.6** demonstrates the changing radii of curvature

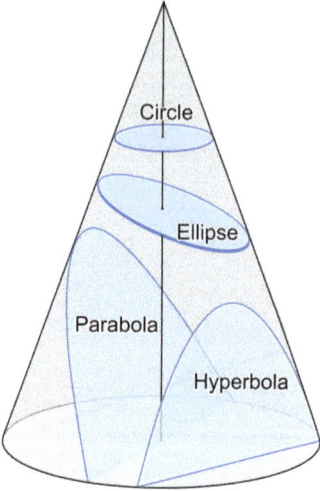

Fig. 9.5: Conic sections

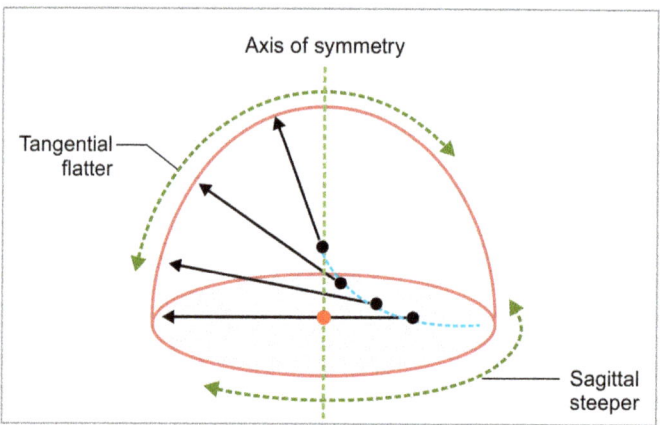

Fig. 9.6: Anatomy of an aspheric surface. This elliptical curve has a radius of curvature that gradually changes away from the centre.

created by rotating an ellipse about an axis of symmetry. When the ellipse is being rotated about the axis of symmetry, it produces a three-dimensional conicoid surface.

For the sake of understanding, we can simplify as under:
- Asphericity is generated by flattening the curve, which introduces astigmatic and power error.
- The peripheral curvature of the aspheric surface, therefore, should ideally change in a manner that neutralizes the effect of such astigmatic and power error, which can be achieved either by steepening of by flattening the peripheral curve.

- For plus lenses, asphericity on front surface requires flattening of curvature away from the center of the lens to minimize the effective gain in oblique power and astigmatic error. Asphericity on the back surface will require steepening of curvature away from center of the lens. The opposite holds true for minus lenses, which can also benefit from asphericity.

Proper base curve selection as recommended by the manufacturer is equally important for aspheric surface also. Even the smaller increments of surface power affect the base curve selection considerably. Consequently, aspheric lenses have more base curve options. Substituting aspheric base curve may have negative effect on the off-axis performance of the lenses. It is interesting to note that actual geometry of aspheric surface helps reduces lens thickness also which is the result of the fact that the sag of an aspheric surface differs from the sag of a spherical surface. At a given diameter, the aspheric surface has shallower sag than spherical surface as shown in **Figure 9.7**. The overall lens looks flatter and thinner as shown in **Figure 9.8**.

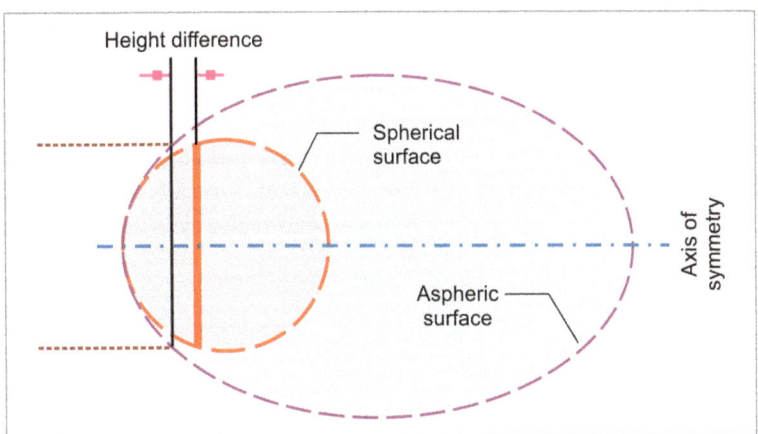

Fig. 9.7: Aspheric versus spherical surface

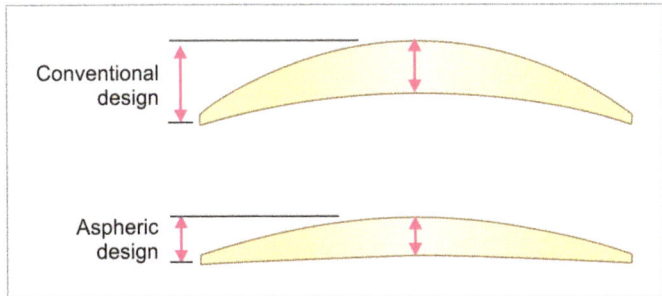

Fig. 9.8: Sagittal depth, conventional versus aspheric lens design

MEASURING AN ASPHERIC SURFACE

Since the curvature of an aspheric surface varies from the center to the periphery, normal measuring instruments cannot measure the front curve value or vertex curvature of an aspheric lens accurately. The manufacturers occasionally publish the design of their lenses, which enables to determine whether the correct design has been supplied. The most common qualitative test to detect whether or not a lens is spherical is to use a lens measure in a sagittal section across the front surface (**Fig. 9.9**). Spherical or toroidal surface will give a constant reading, whereas aspheric surface will vary in power from the center to periphery. However, in low power the change in surface curvature towards the edge of the lens is so subtle that it becomes difficult to verify with the instrument.

PRISM IN ASPHERIC LENSES

The geometric center of the aspheric lens is to be aligned with the optical center of the patient's eyes. This accurate centering of the aspheric lens, throws up an issue with the prescribed prism. Some optical dispensers like to achieve prismatic effect by decentring the lens. Clearly this will move the geometric center of the lens away from the optical axis of the eye which will cause unwanted optical problems for the patient. In order to maintain the alignment of the aspheric geometrical center with the pupil and also have prism in the lens, we need to order the lens with surfaced prism. Typically the lens will have aspheric front side and the rear surface with prism and cylinder surfaced in it.

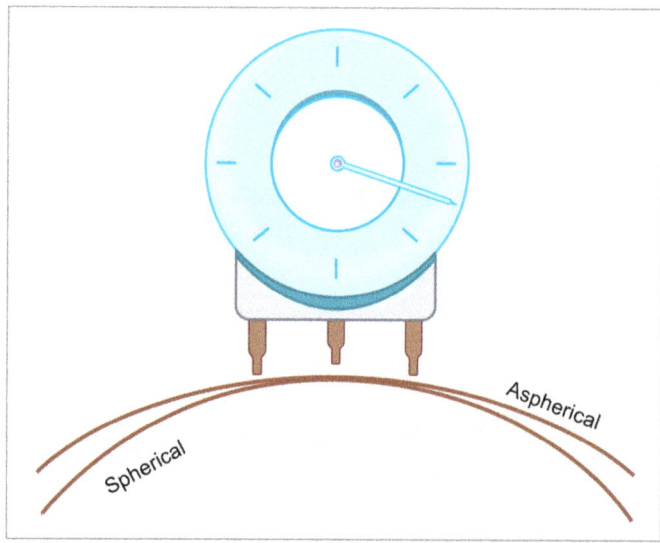

Fig. 9.9: Aspheric surfaces cannot be accurately measured with conventional instruments

However, the true benefit of aspheric lens is achieved only when the optical center of the eye is in alignment with geometric center of the aspheric lens, which is also the pole of the aspheric surface. In a true aspheric lens, asphericity begins right near the center of the lens which also prevents shifting of center to create prism. This suggests grinding prism to decenter the lens is also not the right practice in aspheric lens.

ASPHERIC LENSES FOR APHAKIC PATIENTS

Aphakic spectacle correction requires powers of + 8.00D to + 15.00D. Such a high power correction produces a number of difficulties like:
- Magnification
- Decreased field of view
- Aberration and objects seem swimming in the field of view
- "Popeye" appearance of patients
- Sensitivity to exact position of the lenses.
- Lens weight and thickness.

Various design approaches have been applied to cataract lenses. There are two main approaches the "foveal philosophy" and the "peripheral philosophy". Both use the aspheric curve designing. Foveal philosophy parallels the standard lens design philosophy, trying to give the patient the largest possible dynamic field of view, which is not possible with the spherical curves. Therefore, aspheric curves are used. Peripheral philosophy assumes that aphakics are more of head turner than eye turner. Therefore it uses the front surface curves of diminishing power away from the center to reduce the lens thickness and weight of the lens.

Most of the lens manufacturer offer CR_{39} aspheric lens with convex prolate ellipsoidal surfaces. These series are available in both full aperture and lenticular form, usually with a forty millimetre diameter. They can also be obtained in bifocal forms with round segment and 'D' shapes segment. However, the segment surface itself is not aspherical and since it is cast on ellipsoidal distance portion, the segment tends to be oval shape rather than circular. It is very important while dispensing these high power aspheric lenses that they are carefully centerd both vertically and horizontally, as incorrect centration may well obviate the advantage of the ellipsoidal surface.

Mostly aphakic lenses are made in lenticular design in which central aperture incorporates the optical correction, and is surrounded by a carrier or margin of lower power or even afocal **(Figs. 9.10A to C)**. Natural, sharp and foveal vision is only possible when the wearer views through the aperture. During 1970 aspheric lenses was introduced in which the dividing line between the aperture and margin was blended to make it invisible, Removal of dividing line both improved the appearance of the lenses as well as field of vision by removing the ring scotoma associated with the abrupt change in power at the edge of the aperture.

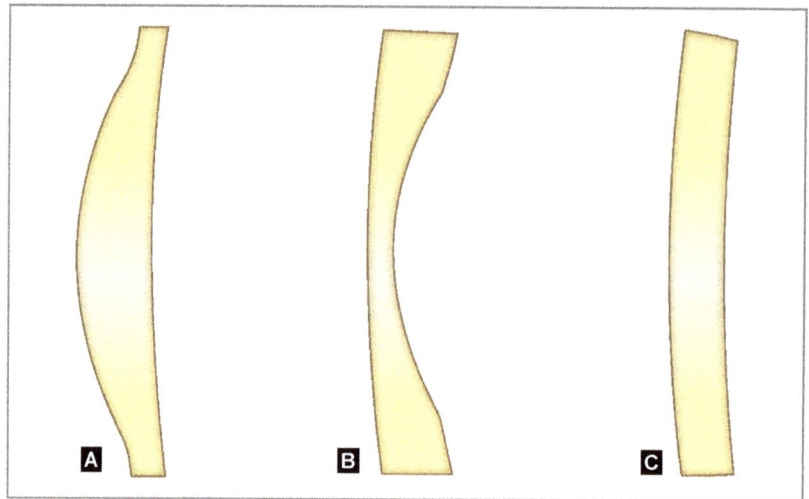

Figs.9.10A to C: (A) Aphakic lens; (B and C) Moulds to manufacture lenticular lens A

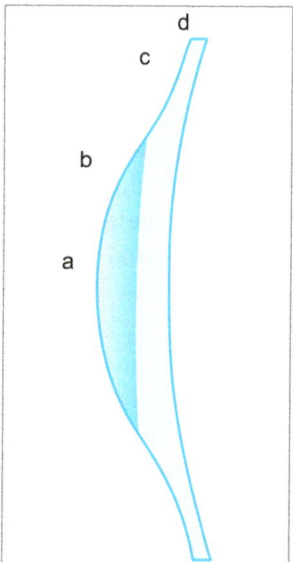

Fig. 9.11: Cataract lens design with convex polynomial surface

With the advent of CNC grinding technology, it became possible to design and manufacture surfaces of almost any complexities. This led the introduction of convex surface that is polynomial form.

For example, in the **Figure 9.11** the zone ab is having the same optical properties on aspheric lens that employs an ellipsoidal surface. It could be free from aberrational astigmatism. Zone bc is seen to be concave in its tangential section. The surface flexes backwards in this region. Since the surface is continuous, there is no annular scotoma between the central ellipsoidal zone and the margin. Zone cd has the same purpose as that of the margin of the lenticular design, i.e. supporting the central aperture.

There are two important advantages: Firstly, the aspheric zone has excellent optical properties, and does not have any aberrational astigmatism of spherical surface. Secondly, the blending is concave which eliminates the ring scotoma that exists at the edges of every plus lens, which is so annoying.

However, today's fact is the aphakic lenses are not much used any more. Implants are almost universal and they allow the use of ordinary correction. A great number of patients go for contact lenses. They need glasses for part time use. A few still have true aphakia, which may take advantage of these lenses.

■ CHECKING LENS POWER IN ASPHERIC LENS

The lens power in case of aspheric lenses can be measured on the focimeter so that it is aligned through the geometric center or middle of aspheric side of the lens. In this area of the lens, the correct power as per the prescription can be seen. As we move away from the geometric center of aspheric surface, the prescription alters—incline with the way the lens surface changes power. The aspheric lens designer specifies a portion, which will be the central region of aspheric side of the lens to be assured of 100% full prescription; the rest of the lens will have a different prescription. The size of this portion depends on the formula, the designer used to formulate the shape of the curves.

■ DISPENSING TIPS

Aspheric lenses represent the ultimate in optics. Using the aspheric curves in a lens, the lens designer provides two benefits—better vision and improved cosmetics. This immediately places the lens into the premium category, providing better profits for every one. This imposes an additional responsibility on dispenser because aspheric can be less forgiving than conventional lenses and requires more precise positioning by the dispenser. A poorly fitted aspheric lens can adversely affect its all benefits. Fitting of aspheric lenses is somewhat similar to the way progressive lenses are fitted **(Fig. 9.12)**.

- **Pupillary distance:** Precise monocular PD measurements position is essential to point the pole of the lens in front of pupil.
- **Vertical height:** The vertical height of each pupil center is marked on the dummy lens of the selected frame.
- **Rotation:** Rotation of the eye must be considered. This requires lowering the optical center based on the pantoscopic angle of the frame. The rule is to lower the optical center 1 mm for every 2 degrees of pantoscopic tilt. However, the maximum drop is 5 mm.

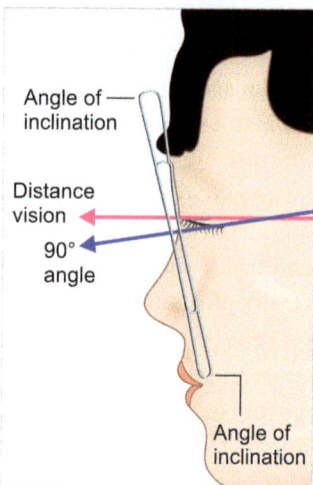

Fig. 9.12: Aspheric fitting guide

Multiple Choice Questions (MCQs)

1. Which of the following is not an advantage of aspheric lenses over spherical lenses?
   a. Aspheric lenses are flatter and thinner
   b. Aspheric lenses provide wider field of clearer vision
   c. Aspheric lenses do not bulge out and thus enhances the cosmetic look of the spectacle
   d. Aspheric lenses enhance the reflection of light

2. Which of the following is true about aspheric lens design?
   a. Front surface of a plus lens becomes flatter away from the center and back surface becomes steeper away from the center.
   b. Front surface of a minus lens becomes steeper away from the center and back surface becomes flatter away from the center.
   c. Surface astigmatism is created to nullify the effect of oblique astigmatism
   d. All of the above

3. Which of the following aberration is corrected by aspheric lens design?
   a. Oblique astigmatism
   b. Chromatic aberration
   c. Comatic aberration
   d. Spherical aberration

Chapter 9: Aspheric Lenses

4. Which of the following is used to denote the degree of asphericity of its surface?
   a. Dioptre
   b. E-value
   c. Curvature
   d. Radius

5. Which of the following is critical for dispensing aspheric lenses?
   a. Always dispense with anti-reflection coating to prevent surface reflection.
   b. Monocular PD measurements is essential to place the pole of the lens in front of pupil
   c. Degree of asphericity should be selected based on the focal power of the lens
   d. All of the above

Answers				
1. d	2. d	3. a	4. b	5. d

Chapter 10

Bifocal Lenses

Eyes age along with rest of us and vision stealing problem becomes more troublesome beginning in the middle age. Usually around the age of 40 years, when a person is found squinting at the newsprint held at the arm's length, he has achieved the middle age milestone: *the arrival of presbyopia*. A presbyopic subject requires a separate correction for distance and near vision, the two prescriptions may be provided as one pair of spectacle in the form of a bifocal lens. A bifocal lens is defined as having two portions of different focal power. The area of the lens used for distance vision is called Distance portion or DP and the area used for near vision is called the Near Portion or Reading Portion or NP. The larger of these two portions is referred to as the main lens (the exception being the up curve bifocal).

The first recorded mention of bifocal spectacle lens is a letter written by Benjamin Franklin in 1784 in which he described a pair of spectacles incorporating such lenses. These were made by the relatively crude method of splitting a distance and a near lens, then mounting the top half of the distance and the bottom half of the near together and were fitted edge-to-edge in a single rim as shown in **Figure 10.1**.

This approach is still in use for prescriptions that cannot be manufactured using mass production technique, an example being where a large amount of prism is required at near but not at distance. Following Franklin's invention, the bifocal lens evolved through a number of stages before the development of

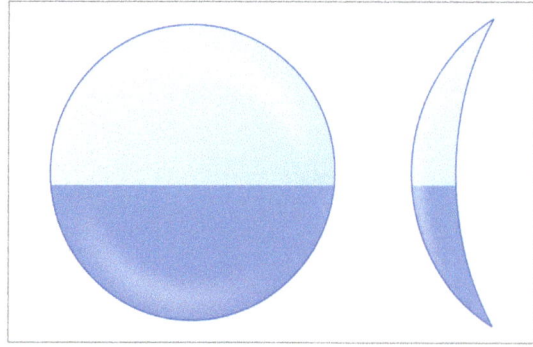

Fig. 10.1: Split bifocal (Franklin design)

modern fused and one-piece bifocal lenses early in this century. Modern version is cosmetically and mechanically improved to suit the mass production also.

TYPES OF BIFOCAL LENSES

Bifocal lenses can be obtained in four basic constructional types as shown in **Flowchart 10.1**.

Fused Bifocal

The first fused bifocal was the fused kryptok invented by Borsch in the year 1908. In countries, where glass lens still represent a sizeable section of the market, the fused bifocal remains the most common form of bifocal design. The round segment is still in production for some markets but no doubt, the most commonly used segments are D-shaped flat top or the C-shaped curved top as shown in **Figure 10.2**.

The segment is permanently bonded onto the convex surface of the lens by heat fusion process and the required addition depends upon:
- The refractive indices of the two glass materials.
- The depression curve.
- The curve worked on the segment side of the lens.

To fuse a segmented bifocal, a countersink cavity is produced on the front surface or the convex side of the crown lens having a refractive index of 1.523 **(Fig. 10.3)**. A flint glass of high refractive index usually of 1.654 is taken. The front surface of the flint button is simply left and a predetermined contact surface is worked on the rear surface of the button to match the curve on the crown blank.

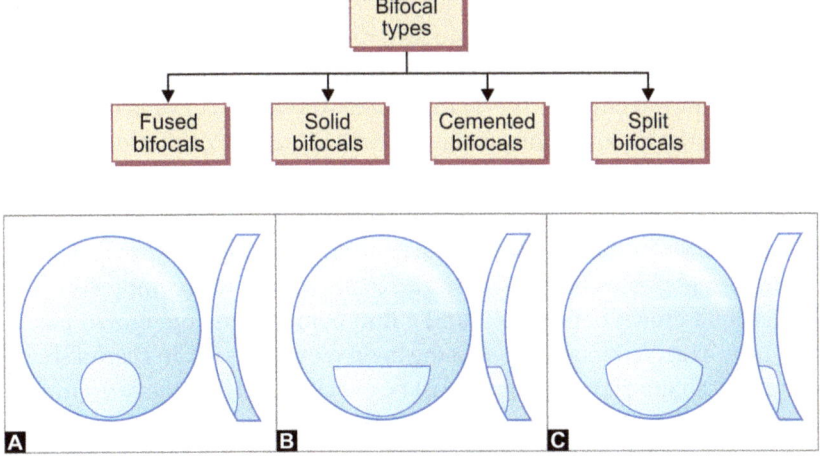

Flowchart 10.1: Types of bifocal lenses

Figs. 10.2A to C: Fused bifocal design: (A) Round segment, (B) D segment flat top, (C) C segment curved top

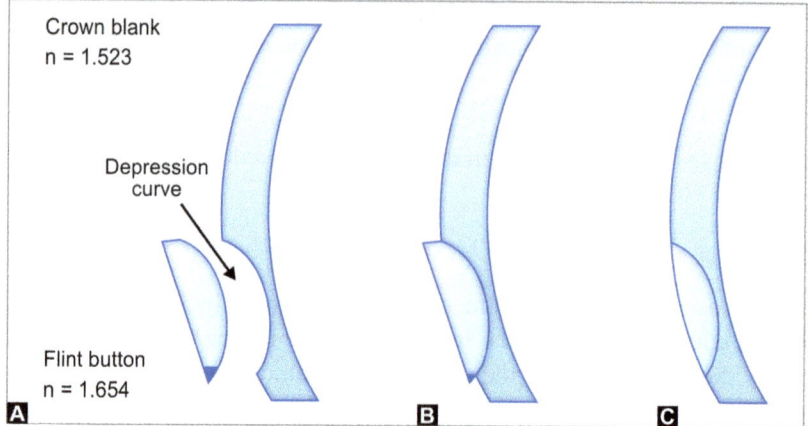

Figs. 10.3A to C: Construction of fused bifocal: (A) Components prior to fusing; (B) Rough fused blank; (C) Semi-finished fused blank

The curve on the contact surface of the button is deliberately made some 0.25D to 0.50D steeper than the depression curve on the corresponding crown blanks so that initially, contact is only made at the center of the curves. The button is placed on the depressed crown portion and the assembled components are then placed on a carborundum block, the surface of which has been molded to match the curve on the back of the crown glass major and the blocks are then kept into the furnace. At around 640ºC the button softens and sags under its own weight, gradually expelling air towards the wire feeler. The steeper curve on the button aids this procedure by tending to unroll the depression curve towards the feeler. Eventually, the whole surface of the button is in contact with the depression curve except for two very small areas around the supporting wires. The resultant fused blanks are then put into rigorous inspection. If, by chance, some dust has remained between the surfaces, a bubble is formed, which may result in rejection of the blank. Since, the front curve is continuous over the distance and near portion; the dividing line of the fused bifocal segment cannot be felt.

Shaped bifocals like D segments, B segments, C segments and curve top bifocals can be produced by means of composite buttons, made up of two or three different glasses **(Fig. 10.4)**. In each of these cases the composite button consists of a crown component and a flint component. The crown portion must have exact refractive index as the main crown glasses. In case of shaped bifocal, the shape of the segment must be checked and if necessary it must be corrected so that it has the required segment diameter and segment depth. This can be achieved by grinding a small amount of vertical prism relative to the segment side surface.

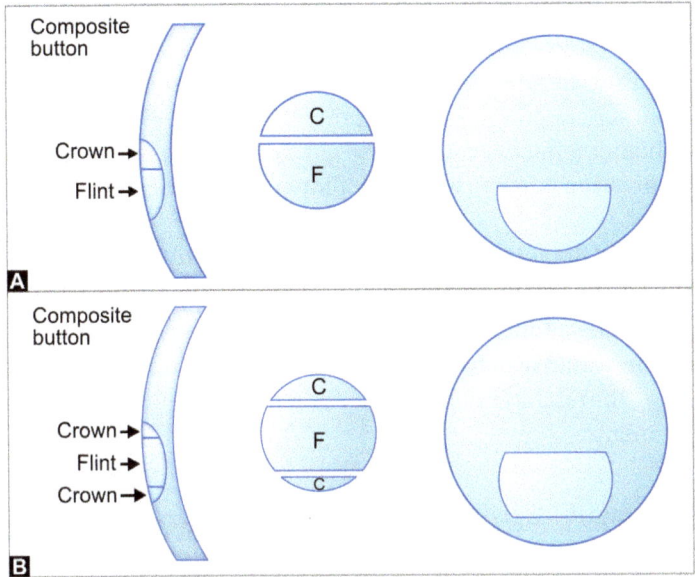

Figs. 10.4A and B: Composite buttons for different bifocal shapes: (A) D-segment flat top bifocal; (B) B-segment

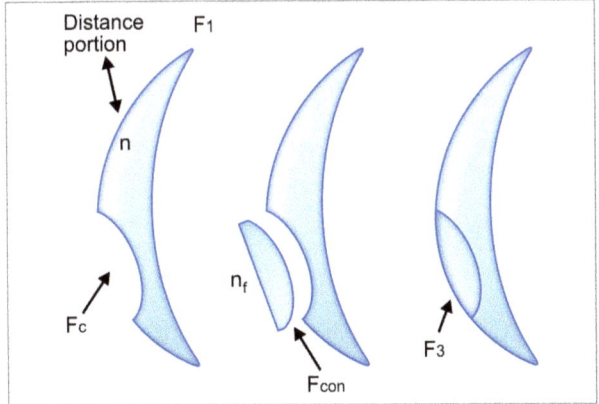

Fig. 10.5: Stages to manufacture round segment bifocal

Reading Addition of a Fused Bifocal

The fused bifocal is produced by fusing a higher index flint to the main crown glass as shown in **Figure 10.5**. A countersink cavity having a specific depression curve is made onto the convex side of the crown glass whereon the flint is fused at a high temperature. If we can find out the curvature required for the countersink cavity, we can determine the resultant addition. The following factors determine the addition:

- The refractive index of the crown glass, denoted by n and the refractive index of the flint glass denoted by n_f.
- The front surface power of the distance portion of the crown glass, say F_1.
- The front surface power over the segment area, say F_3 which is greater owing to the higher refractive index of the glass of the segment.
- The depression curve to which the flint button is fused has a power in air, say Fc.
- The power of the contact surface of the button in situ denoted by F_{con}, which also forms the part of the total addition.

Therefore, the addition from the front surface would be $(F_3 - F_1)$. But the total addition would also be affected by the contact surface of the button in situ, i.e., F_{con}. The total addition for near A, therefore, would be the sum of these two components:

$$A = (F_3 - F_1) + F_{con}$$

The quantity $(F_3 - F_1)$ is the function of the refractive indices of the respective materials and hence can be shown to be equal to $F_1 (n_f - n)/(n - 1)$. Similarly, F_{con} can be shown to be equal to $- Fc (n_f - n)/(n - 1)$.

Substituting the values:

$$A = F_1\left(\frac{n_f - n}{n - 1}\right) - F_c\left(\frac{n_f - n}{n - 1}\right)$$

Or, $\quad A = F_1(K) - F_c(K)$

Or, $\quad A = K(F_1 - F_c)$

Or, $\quad A/K = F_1 - F_c$

Or, $\quad F_c = F_1 - A/K$

∴ $\quad F_c = F_1 - A\left(\dfrac{n-1}{n_f - n}\right)$

Example:

(1) Consider a lens with F_1 of + 6.00D and refractive index of 1.523 and 1.654 for n and n_f respectively. If required addition is + 2.00, then

$F_c = 6 - (0.523/0.131)\,2$

$= - 1.98D$

Solid Bifocal

Solid bifocal can be considered as one piece bifocal, made from single piece of material. They can be made by molding or casting one surface and working the other (usually plastics), by molding or casting both the surfaces (almost always plastics) or by working both the surfaces (almost always glass). Most segment shapes and sizes, from E style to round are available as solid plastic bifocals. Blended bifocals are solid, usually round segment bifocals in which the segment edge blends into the distance portion.

The reading addition of a solid bifocal is obtained by raising a second curve on one surface of the lens to form the segment. The segment can be worked on either side of the lens **(Fig. 10.6)**. The surface on the segment side of the lens that forms the part of the distance power is called the DP surface and the power of this surface is referred to as the DP curve. The raised curve on the segment side that forms the near power is called the segment surface and its power is known as RP curve. The reading addition is the difference between the RP curve and the DP curve. Thus, if the segment is on the convex surface of the lens and the DP curve is + 6.00D and the RP curve is + 8.00D, the reading addition would be + 2.00D. Alternatively, if the segment is situated on the concave side of the lens and the DP curve is – 6.00D, then to produce a reading addition of + 2.00D, the RP curve would have to be – 4.00D.

Cemented Bifocal

A segment is glued onto the surface of a single vision lens **(Fig. 10.7)**. Theoretically, almost any prescription can be obtained and it is also possible to get almost any shape of segment, in any position on the main lens. Traditionally they are made from glasses but they can be made from plastic materials too. Until about 1960, the adhesive in common use was Canada balsam—a resin exuded by the balsam fir tree. Canada balsam was easy to apply and reapply, but its adhesive is deteriorated after being subjected to mechanical, thermal or chemical shock. More recently, ultraviolet cured epoxy resins have replaced Canada balsam and provide excellent long-term adhesion of glass components.

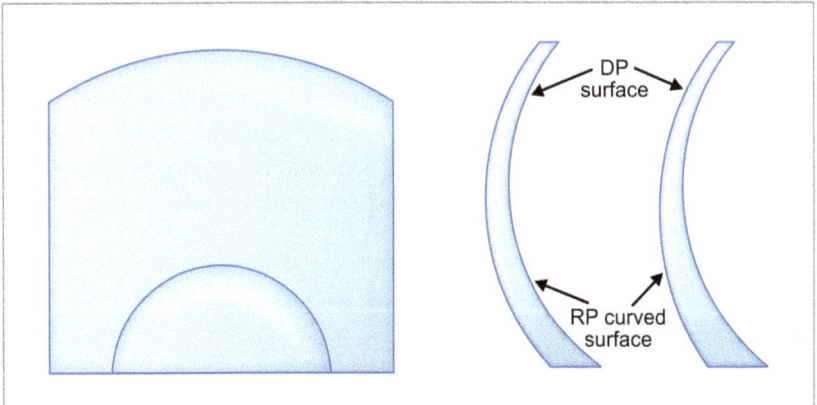

Fig. 10.6: The solid bifocal in which the reading addition is the difference between the RP curve and the DP curve. The segment can be worked either on the concave surface or on the convex surface

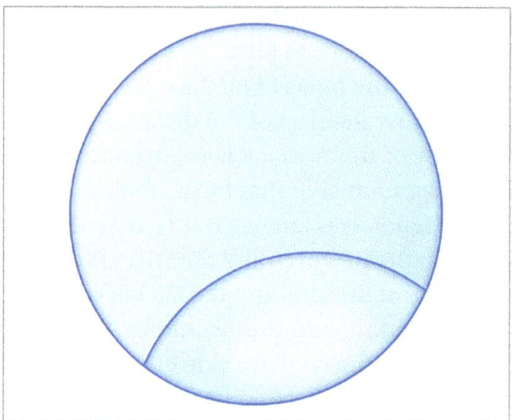

Fig.10.7: Cemented bifocal

Split Bifocal

Also known as Franklin bifocal lenses is made of two separate lenses held together by the frame. They are almost invariably an E-style bifocal, although very rarely they are made as very large segment diameter in down curve forms. They sometimes have their two sections bonded together and they can be made in either glass or plastic materials. Unfortunately, dirt tends to accumulate in the joint between the lenses, however well made they are and no matter how careful the subject is in cleaning them.

■ BIFOCAL SEGMENT SHAPES

The most commonly available Bifocal shapes are depicted in **Flowchart 10.2**. Segments vary from tiny "B segment" to "E-style" in which the whole bottom half of the lens is used for near portion. Historically, there were huge number of segment shapes with minor variations and corresponding number of descriptions used for them. But now the apparent choice has reduced, so that a small number of terms can be used to cover all multifocals. The most popular bifocal shape at present in common use is probably D-segment, E-style and round segment bifocal. B-segment and C-segment are relatively rare, while any other shape is almost unheard of.

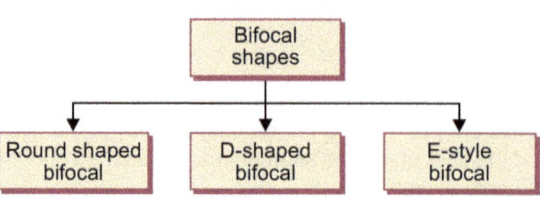

Flowchart 10.2: Popular shapes bifocal lenses

Round Shaped Bifocal

Round segment bifocal have a segment with a dividing line that is a single circular arc which is least visible compared to the other bifocals. When placed at the bottom half of the lens, they are often called "down curve" bifocal. The center of the segment in round shape bifocal fall much below from the top, so they must be fitted a little higher than the other bifocals. This gives rise to "jump" at the edge of the segment when the line of gaze passes from distance to near.

The kryptok bifocal is one of the most popular round bifocals **(Fig. 10.8)**. The design as developed by John L Borsch Jr, in 1908 made use of distance lens of crown and a segment lens of flint glass. The process involved fusing of flint glass into a countersink curve made on the convex side of the crown lens under a high temperature. If the heat is not carefully controlled during the fusing operation, the countersink curve will warp and will produce unwanted optical aberration.

The round Barium (Nokrome) bifocal differs from the kryptok bifocal in the use of high index barium glass for the segment instead of flint glass and in the close matching of the countersink curve and the rear surface of the button. Close matching of curves cuts down on the heat required for fusing process. This in turn results in more accurate curves and better lenses.

Round segment bifocal, especially those with low power having small segments are among the least conspicuous of conventional bifocals. Only the cosmetic or blended bifocals and the progressive addition lenses are less conspicuous multifocals.

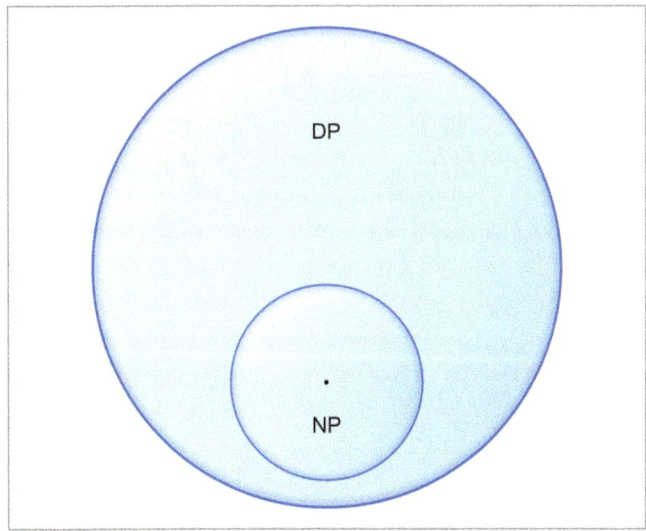

Fig. 10.8: Round segment bifocal

D-Shaped Bifocal

D segment bifocals are available in solid plastics and fused glass forms. They are a nice compromise lens, giving a relatively wide reading area at the point of visual entry into the segment, with less of a thickness problem than E-style. Cosmetically, the straight edge of D segment **(Fig. 10.9A)** is little more noticeable and therefore cosmetically less attractive to many patients, than edge of round segment. There is still some jump at the edge of most D segments, although it is less than round segments. A modified shape of D shape bifocal is C segments which are also available with a slight rounded top instead of flat tops **(Fig. 10.9B)**. The principle advantage of C segments over D segments is probably in glazing and surfacing. Minor errors made in the cylinder axis during surfacing can be glazed to the correct axis and they can be far less noticeable. B segments are like a D bifocal with the bottom chopped off **(Fig. 10.9C)**. Losing the top of the circle, as with the D-shaped bifocal, reduces the jump at the edge of the segment and losing the bottom gets rid of the area which is potentially the worst optically and thereby allows a clear view of the feet through the bottom.

E-Style Bifocal

E-style bifocal is one-piece bifocal lens with two different curves ground usually on the front surface **(Fig. 10.10)**. The optical center of both the distance and

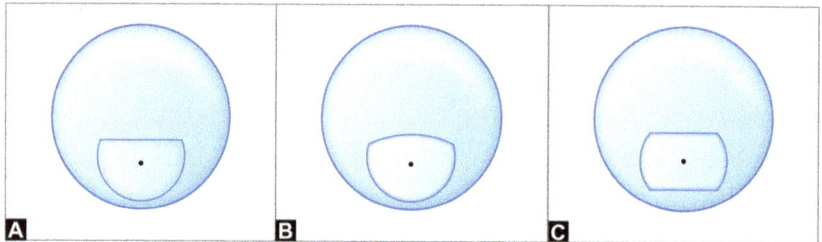

Figs. 10.9A to C: (A) Straight top D bifocal, (B) Curve top bifocal, (C) B segment bifocal.
The dot indicates the geometric center of the segment

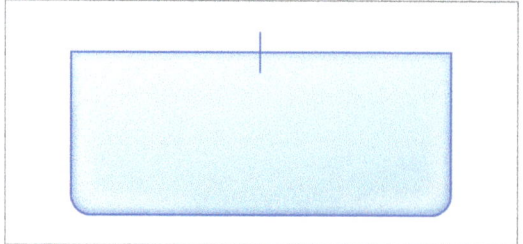

Fig. 10.10: E-style bifocal. The cross shows the position of optical center

the near lens lie on the dividing line. It is, therefore, classified as monocentric bifocal. The difference in curves between the distance and the near portion of the lens produces a ledge that is most prominent towards the outer edge of the lens. E-style bifocals, popularly known as executive bifocal are invariably solid bifocal. Most of optical center of the distance and near portion on the dividing line gets rid of vertical image jump.

To locate the segment center, hold the lens 4 to 5 inches away from a straight line and move the lens from left to right, the straight line will break as it passes from the upper portion of the lens to the segment. At the segment center point, the straight line will have the continuity as shown in the **Figure 10.11**.

The big advantage of E-style bifocal is that the entire bottom half of the lens is for near vision. Thickness can be a problem in hypermetropic prescription. Because of the fact that both distance and near optical center fall on the dividing line, the thickness of the finished lens is largely controlled by the resultant near prescription rather than the distance prescription. Hence, + 3.00D with + 3.00D addition would have a center thickness equivalent to + 6.00D, i.e. for a plus prescription the center thickness is equivalent to the reading addition plus the distance power. The edge thickness can be comparable to – 3.00D, i.e. the difference between distance prescription and the resultant near prescription. Prism thinning can reduce but can never eliminate the effect.

Contrarily, in minus lens the center thickness is affected by less power than the distance prescription, i.e. if the distance prescription is – 4.00D and the near addition is + 2.00D, then the sum of distance power and the near addition is – 2.00D. So, the center thickness can be comparable to – 2.00D. Prism thinning can improve the appearance of the top edge **(Figs. 10.12 and 10.13)**.

Another problem associated with the type of bifocal lens is the reflection from the top edge of the straight top bifocal which can be annoying to the patient **(Fig. 10.14)**. Reflection from this edge can often be seen by others, making the segment more obvious to others.

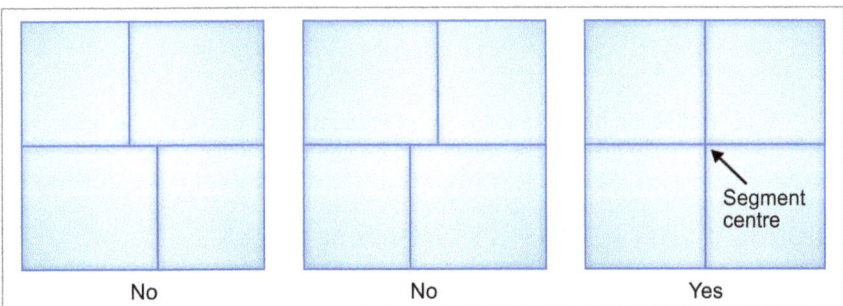

Fig. 10.11: The segment center of E-style bifocal is at the point where the straight vertical line will have continuity

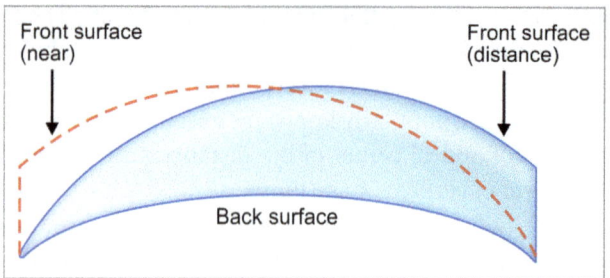

Fig. 10.12: Section through the common optical centers of distance and near areas of an E-style bifocal in case of plus prescription

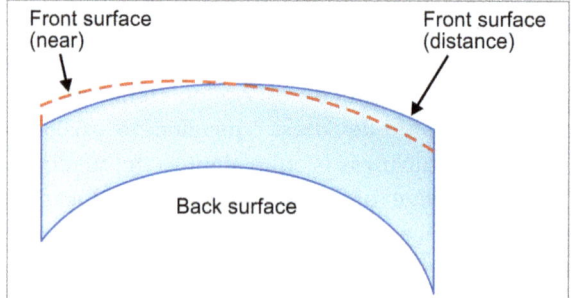

Fig. 10.13: Section through the common optical centers of distance and near areas of an E-style bifocal in case of minus prescription

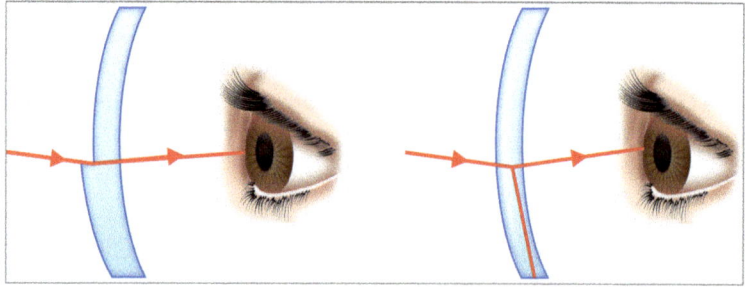

Fig. 10.14: Reflection from the top edge of straight top bifocals can be annoying to the patient. It can also be seen by others

OPTICAL CHARACTERISTICS OF BIFOCAL LENSES

Optical characteristics of bifocal lenses vary widely from one bifocal lens type to another, so they should be taken into consideration when selecting a bifocal segment type for a given patient. The common difficulties that are associated with different types of bifocal lenses are shown in **Flowchart 10.3**.

Flowchart 10.3: Optical characteristics of bifocal lenses

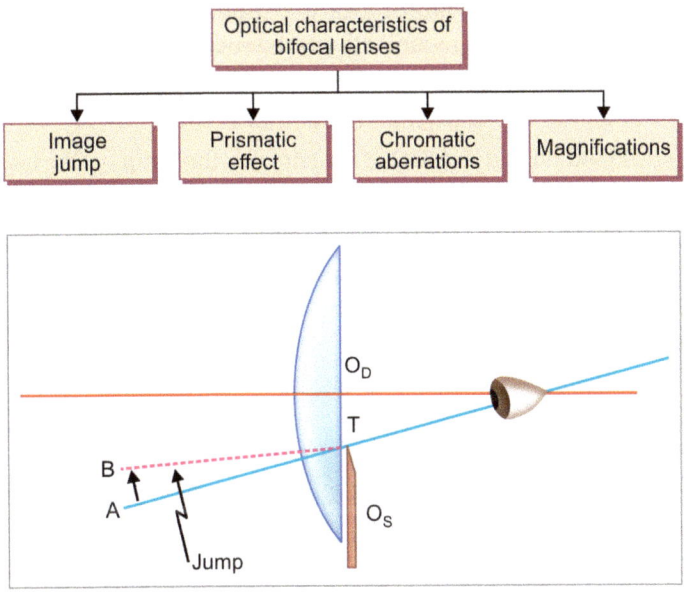

Fig. 10.15: Jump at the bifocal dividing line

Image Jump

When looking from distance portion to the near portion of a bifocal lens, the sudden change in the prismatic effect because of the introduction of the base down prism by the segment causes the world to "jump". This displacement of the patient's visual world can be very disturbing and often dangerous particularly with steps and kerbs. It has both vertical and horizontal element. Jump occurs all around the edge of the bifocal segment, although it is at the top part which is most frequently noticed.

The base of the prism lies at the optical center of the segment Os. Consider the eye viewing through the distance portion. As the gaze is lowered, the eye encounters an ever increasing prismatic effect as it rotates away from the optical center of the distance portion **(Fig. 10.15)**. When the eye enters the near portion, it suddenly encounters the base down prism exerted by the segment at the segment top. The effect is twofold. Firstly, object that lies in the direction of AT, appears to lie in the direction BT. Apparently, they have jumped to a new position. Secondly, light from the angular zone BTA, around the edge of the segment, cannot enter the eye. The segment dividing line causes an annular scotoma within which the object is completely hidden until the wearer moves his head to shift the zone in which jump occurs.

The amount of jump is simply the magnitude of the prismatic effect exerted by the segment at its dividing line that is the product of the distance from the segment top to the segment optical center, in centimeters and the power of the reading addition. For a round bifocal the distance from the segment top to the optical center of the segment is simply the segment radius and therefore, for circular segments:

Jump = Segment radius in cms × reading addition.

But for shaped bifocal like B, C or D segments, the jump will be less as it is:

Jump = Reading addition × Distance to the center of the circle of which the segment is part from the top edge **(Fig. 10.16)**.

For most of the E-style bifocal, with their distance and near optical centers coinciding at the dividing line, the jump is purely horizontal at points away from the common center **(Fig. 10.17)**.

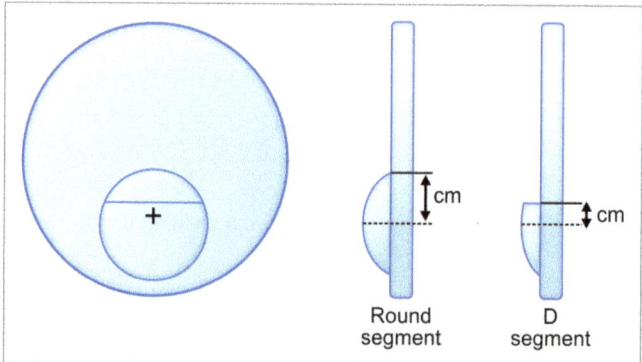

Fig. 10.16: Image jump at the top of round segment due to the segment alone is the product of the addition power and the radius of the segment in centimeters. For a shaped bifocal, say 'D' segment the prismatic effect at the top edge is the distance of the top edge from the center of the circle of which the segment is the part multiplied by the addition

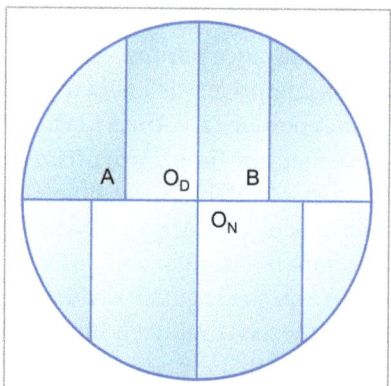

Fig. 10.17: Lateral jump in an E-style bifocal. Line at the optical center is undeviated. But vertical lines at A and B show a lateral displacement at the segment top

Clearly the jump is completely independent of the power of the main lens and the position of the distance optical center. Jump increases as the distance from the segment top to the segment optical center increases, i.e. in case of round segments as the segment diameter increases.

For example, if the reading addition is + 2.00D, the jump exerted by a 24 mm segment is 2.4 Δ BD in case of round segment bifocal.

But in case of D segment where segment size is, say, 28 x 19 and the segment center lies just 5 mm below the segment top, the jump will be only 1.00Δ BD. Reduced jump is probably the one reason why shaped bifocal have proved to be so popular.

To eliminate the jump effect in a bifocal lens, it is necessary to work the segment in such a fashion that its optical center coincides with the segment top.

Prismatic Effect

When a wearer uses single vision lens and he gazes downward to read through the lens, he encounters a prismatic effect. The prismatic effect will change in the near visual zone when he wears a bifocal lens. While determining the prismatic effect in the near portion, it is to be understood that bifocal lenses are made of two separate components—a main lens with a distance prescription and a supplementary segment lens with a power equal to reading addition.

The optical center of the main lens, i.e., distance optical center is referred to as O_D and the optical center of the segment lens as O_s. The total power of the near portion is the sum of the distance portion power and the reading addition of the lens and the prismatic effect at some point in the near portion is given by the sum of the prismatic effect of the distance portion and the prismatic effect of the segment lens.

Consider a case of round shape bifocal lens as depicted in **Figure 10.18** the prismatic effect at the NVP, 8 mm below the distance optical center and 5 mm below the segment top can be determined as follows:

The prismatic effect at 8 mm below the optical center in + 3.00D lens can be found out from the decent ration relationship P = cf, where C is the decent ration in centimeters and F is the power of the lens.

Hence, P = 0.8 × 3.00
 = 2.4Δ BU

The segment would exert base down prism at the NVP which can be deduced as follows:

Suppose the segment diameter is 38 mm. The distance from the dividing line to the optical center of the segment is 38/2 or 19 mm. Since, NVP lies 5 mm below the segment top, it must lie 14 mm above the segment center. Hence, the prism from segment is:

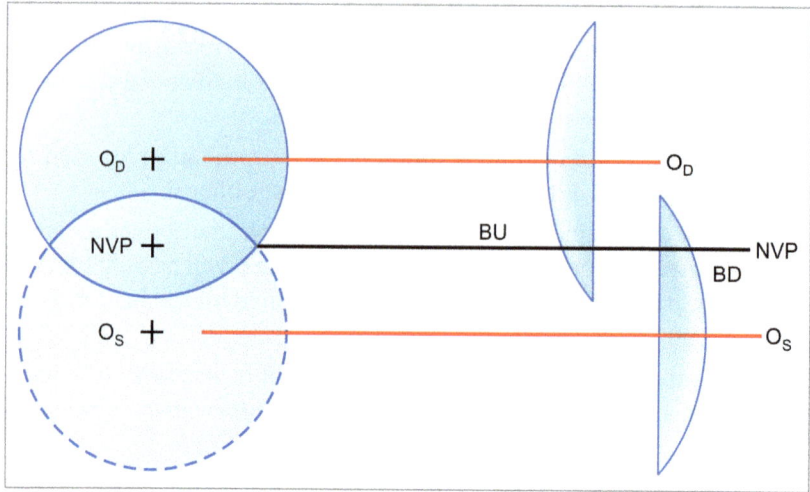

Fig. 10.18: Prismatic effects at the near visual point (NVP) of a bifocal lens. O_D is the optical center of the distance portion. O_s is the optical center of the segment lens

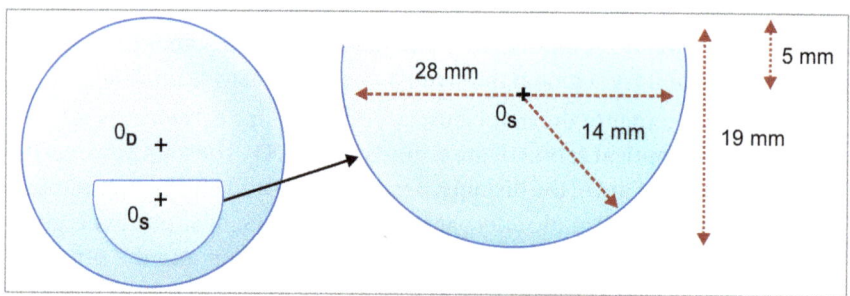

Fig. 10.19: D-shaped segment of 28 × 19. O_s is the optical center of segment which lies 5 mm below the segment top and coincides with NVP

P = 1.4 × 2.00
 = 2.8 Δ BD.

The total prismatic effect at the NVP is the sum of 2.4Δ BU and 2.8Δ BD, which is 0.4Δ BD.

Now, consider a case of D-shape bifocal as shown in **Figure 10.19**. In this case D shape segment size of 28 × 19 mm has been prescribed. If we assume that NVP is located in exactly the same position 8 mm below the O_D and 5 mm below the segment top. The optical center of the segment O_s now coincides with the NVP, so segment adds no prism at this point. So the net prismatic effect would be only 2.4Δ BU, what is exerted by distance portion. This is an important advantage of the shaped bifocal.

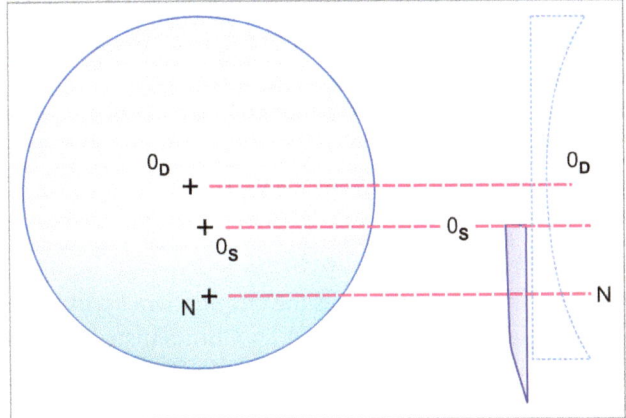

Fig. 10.20: E-style bifocal. The segment exerts base up prism at the NVP

In case of E-style bifocal, the optical center of the segment is positioned on the dividing line which is above the NVP and since the power of the segment is positive, the segment will exert base up prism **(Fig. 10.20)**. If we assume that NVP is located at the same position, i.e. 5 mm below the optical center of the segment or the segment top, the prismatic effect would be:

P = 0.5 x 2.00
 = 1.0Δ BU

The prismatic effect due to the distance lens would be:

P = 0.5 × 3.00
 = 1.5Δ BU

The total prismatic effect would be 2.5Δ BU.

In case of minus power, the distance portion will exert base down prism. Consequently the prismatic effect will change depending upon the type of the segment shape. E-style bifocal will exert least prismatic effect in minus power. In case of straight top D shape bifocal which has an optical center coinciding with the NVP, the vertical prismatic effect at reading level is due to the distance power only. Therefore, it does not change when the wearer switches from single vision to bifocal lens. The total vertical prismatic effect at the reading level is of practical importance as it determines the amount of transverse chromatic aberration the wearer will be subjected to.

Chromatic Aberration

Transverse Chromatic Aberration (TCA) arising out of the oblique rays is the potential problem for the wearer of the single vision lenses as well as bifocal lenses. The effect of TCA is the colour fringes to be seen surrounding the image of the high contrast targets, while looking through a point in the lens away from its optical center. As a result of the fact that bifocal segment is viewed through the edge of the distance lens, problems can arise due to TCA arising from the distance vision prismatic effect. When the prismatic effect at a point is known, the TCA at that point can be found by dividing the prismatic effect by the Abbe Number for the material which is denoted by V, i.e.

TCA = P/V

(Where, P stands for the prismatic effect).

This paraxial relationship expresses the chromatism in prism dioptres and the average threshold value is in order of 0.1Δ. Chromatism less than this value are unlikely to give rise to complaints. In case of solid bifocals including both glass and plastic, the chromatism can be found simply by dividing the total prismatic effect at the point in question by the Abbe Number for the material. Thus, in case of solid bifocal of + 5.00D with reading addition + 2.00D, made with a 24 mm diameter segment and a segment drop of 2mm, the vertical prismatic effect at a point 6 mm below the segment top is given by:

$$P = cf$$
Or, $$P = 0.8 \times 5$$
Or, $$P = 4.00\Delta \text{ BU}$$

The prismatic effect due to segment is:

$$P = cf$$
Or, $$P = 0.6 \times 2$$
Or, $$P = 1.2\Delta \text{ BD}$$

So, the total prismatic effect would be 2.8" Base Up, the horizontal prismatic effect being ignored. Therefore, TCA at this point would be, if the material is CR_{39} with Abbe number 58:

$$\begin{align} TCA &= P/V \\ &= 2.8 / 58 \\ &= 0.05\Delta \end{align}$$

This value at the center of the near visual zone is unlikely to cause any complaints.

In case of fused bifocal in which the near portion combines a crown glass element with a flint glass element of lower abbe value, the chromatism is the sum of three components—distance element, chromatism because of depression curve and chromatism due to segment element. The distance element of crown glass represents the power of the distance portion and is denoted by F, the centered depression curve, also a part of crown glass, is denoted by $-Ak$, where A is the reading addition and k is the blank ratio $(n-1)/(n_s - n)$. The power of the segment element is given by $A(k+1)$.

At a point N, in the near portion, three components contribute to the prismatic effect and hence to the chromatism at that point. Two components are made from crown glass and the third is the flint glass element of the near portion. If the distance from the distance optical center to the point N is denoted by Y and the distance from N to segment optical center to N by Ys which must be given a minus sign when Os lies below N. Then chromatism at point N is given by:

$$TCA = y(F/V) - \{(-ys)(AK/V)\} + \left\{(-ys)\left(\frac{A[K+1]}{Vs}\right)\right\}$$

Where V = Abbe value of crown glass
Vs = Abbe value of flint segment
k = $(n-1)/(n_s - n)$

So, in our above example:
Y = 0.8 Ys = 0.6
F = 5.00 A = 2.0
V = 58 Vs = 36 (say).
K = $(n-1)/(n_s - n)$ = 1.523 - 1 / 1.654 - 1.523 = 4.

Putting up the values:

$$TCA = 0.8\left(\frac{5}{58}\right) - \left\{(-06)\left(\frac{2\times 4}{58}\right)\right\} + \left\{(-0.6)\left(\frac{2[4+1]}{36}\right)\right\}$$

$= (0.8 \times 0.086) - \{(0.6)(0.38)\} + \{(-0.8)(0.278)\}$

$= (0.0688) - (-0.0828) + (-0.167)$

$= -0.02\Delta$

This is negligible.

Once again the flat top fused bifocal demonstrates its superiority over round segment, since the distance Ys is negligible in case of most shaped bifocal.

Magnification

Another consequence of the reading addition is the small magnification difference between the distance and the reading portion. Patient may be aware of this, although it is unlikely to cause serious problems as the size change occurs in both eyes. This may give rise to change in perceived distance rather than aniseikonia.

We have seen that a bifocal free of jump (executive type) will induce a certain amount of prismatic effect at the reading level; while the bifocal that induces no prismatic effect at the reading level (straight top shaped bifocal) is subject to a certain amount of jump. For the long term spectacle wearer who is already accustomed to a certain amount of prismatic effect, this will change when bifocal lenses are first worn. Adaptation to this new type of prismatic effect should not be difficult. However, jump manifests itself each time the wearer directs his line of vision downwards across the dividing line. Even if the patient will learn to ignore the displacement of his environment, it will never cease to occur. Consequently, we should expect jump to be a greater problem for the wearer than the segment induced prismatic effect.

PRISM CONTROLLED BIFOCALS

Bifocal designs that permit control of the prismatic effects in the near portion by the incorporation of prism in the segment are known as prism controlled bifocals. Prismatic effect at any point in the near portion depends upon the power of the main lens and the power of the segment lens, and the positions of their individual optical centers in relation to the visual point at which we wish to find the prismatic effect. Sometimes it is necessary to alter the prismatic effect at the NVP, for example to balance the vertical prismatic effects at the NVP or to provide horizontal prism correction in the reading portion only. This can be achieved by using a bifocal design for which the method of construction allows independent centration of the reading portion. Such a design is called a Prism controlled bifocals. This kind of bifocal design is constructed to incorporate the prism in the segment and is totally independent of any prism included in the main lens. There are several methods by which prism may be incorporated in the near segment only. They are shown in the **Flowchart 10.4.**

Split Bifocal

Two half lenses – one for distance and another for reading are made from two separate lenses for which the power and centration may be chosen at will. Reading portion carries the corrective vertical prism. Full prism control is possible in Split bifocals.

Cemented Bifocals

A separate prism segment is attached to the main lens using permanent epoxy resin adhesives.

Flowchart 10. 4: Methods by which prism may be incorporated in the near segment only

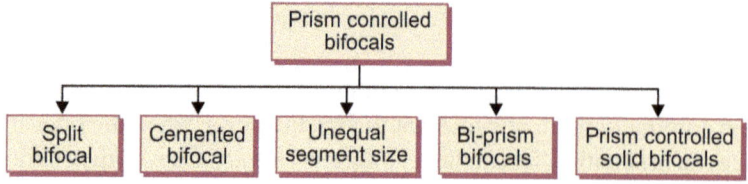

Unequal Segment Sizes

Although, visually a little strange for beholders of those wearing a combination of unequal segment sizes in two eyes, vertical prismatic effect due to anisometropia can be controlled by unequal sizes of the round segment in both the eyes. The heights of top of the segment must be at the same, as when the eyes are depressed from the line of distance vision they must meet the upper margin of the reading portion simultaneously. From Prentice rule, the following expression can be deduced for round segment down curve bifocal:

Difference in segment radii (in cms) x near addition = Amount of relative vertical prism overcome.

Example – RE + 3.00 Dsph

LE + 4.00 Dsph

BE Near Add + 3.00 Dsph

Round bifocal 20 mm segment size.

Upper margin 2 mm below optical center.

Reading point 6 mm below the top edge of segment.

The reading point in the above case is 8 mm below the distance center and 4 mm above the center of the segment.

In the RE, prismatic effect produced by distance correction at this point will be:

$$3 \times 0.8 = 2.4\Delta \text{ BU}.$$

The prismatic effect produced by the segment at this point is:

$$3 \times 0.4 = 1.2\Delta \text{ BD}.$$

Therefore, the resultant prism at this reading point in RE is:

$$1.2\Delta \text{ BU}.$$

Similarly, in LE, the resultant prism is 2.0Δ BU, makes a difference of 0.8Δ BU in LE, which may produce discomfort. To overcome this we have to move the center of the reading segment in the right eye up, to reduce the base down effect and in the left eye, we have to move the center of the reading segment down to increase the base down effect. The difference to be eliminated is 0.8Δ, i.e., 0.4Δ in each eye. The amount, therefore, by which the position of the centers of the segments is to be moved is given by:

$$A \times 3 = 0.4\Delta$$

Therefore, A = 0.4 / 3 = 0.133 cms

Or, A = 1.33 mm

Hence, RE segment will be 17.34 mm diameter and LE segment will be 22.66 mm. A 17 mm segment in right eye and a 23 mm segment in left eye will practically balance the vertical prism at the NVP. Bigger segment will be placed in front of more hyperopic eye or least myopic eye.

In case of shaped segment bifocal, prism control by unequal segment sizes are not useful due to their construction as the optical center of the segment is just around the NVP at which we consider the prismatic effect.

Bi-prism Bifocals

A bi-prism is achieved by surfacing the concave rear surface with the base up prism of equal value to the imbalance between the right and left prescriptions over the entire lens, i.e., distance and reading. Next base down prism with the same amount is worked on the distance curve of the front surface, i.e., on the top part of the lens only. This leaves a lens with zero prisms at distance and base up prism at near **(Figs. 10.21A to E)**.

The result of this entire process creates a horizontal dividing line between the two portions of the lens. For this reason, bi-prism technique is applied to flat top D segments and E-style segments as the bi-prism dividing line can be made to coincide with exactly the top line of the segment. It is usually recommended

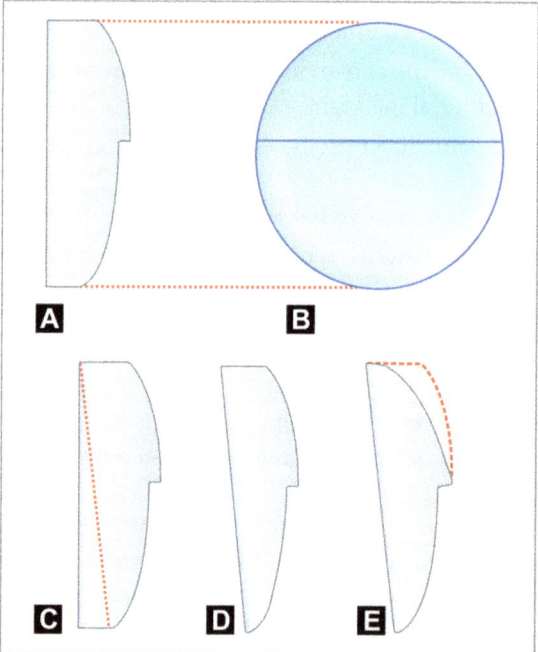

Figs 10.21A to E: Stages in the production of an E-style bi-prism bifocal from the semi-finished lens

(a) Semi-finished lens
(b) Front view
(c) Base up prism is applied across whole of the rear surface
(d) Lens with base up prism
(e) Base down prism is applied to front surface, distance only

that the minimum prism worked is 2Δ in order to obtain a clear dividing line between the two zones. Slab off can only provide a variation in vertical prism and special skill is needed to achieve a neat, straight slab line coinciding with the segment line. Some higher index resins are too soft to produce a clean line, the reason why polycarbonate cannot be slabbed.

Prism Controlled Solid Bifocal

Prism controlled solid bifocal lenses, surely are the most versatile prism segment lens of all, allows to achieve separate control of prismatic elements in both the distance and near portions **(Fig. 10.22)**. Unlike lenses for the control of anisometropia whose correction is only for the vertical prismatic element, a prism controlled solid bifocal lens can correct vertically, horizontally and any oblique angle.

The segment surface of this bifocal saucer blank shows the same axis of revolution as the DP surface, the centration of the reading portion is dependent upon the segment diameter and the prescription of the lens. The segment does not incorporate a separate prismatic effect and is constructed by depressing the reading portion surface below the level of the DP surface and dropping a prism into the depression. The apical angle of this prism is the same angle as that which the blank must rotate through to obtain the prescribed prism in the segment.

Truly this is very interesting lens which provides a comfortable binocular vision to many who otherwise would only achieve monocular vision or revert to two pairs of single vision lenses.

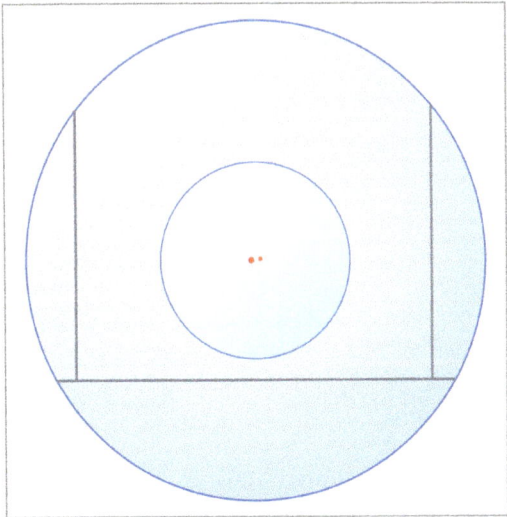

Fig. 10.22: Cutting of solid bifocal disk to obtain one semi-finished segment blank

INVISIBLE BIFOCALS

Invisible bifocals are one-piece bifocal lenses having round segment, in which the line of demarcation between the distance portion of the lens and the bifocal segment has been obliterated by a polishing process **(Fig. 10.23)**. The result is an invisible bifocal segment. Optically the lens performs the same as a standard round shaped bifocal, as only two actual zones of focus exist – one for distance and one for near. The obliteration process produces distortion around the bifocal segment which varies in width from less than 3 mm to just under 5 mm, depending on the power of the near addition and the base curve. This area serves as the boundary of the segment and permits the lens to be fitted according to the same provisions that affect an ordinary round bifocal. Since the blending is wider than the actual demarcation line, the bifocal may require either slightly higher placement of the top of the segment or greater depression of the gaze for reading. The manufacturer recommends fitting this bifocal 1 mm higher than other types of bifocals. The invisible bifocals only cater to the wearer's vanity. Some bifocal wearers are ready to accept the blurred area and the comparatively small reading field in order to avoid the stigma of wearing bifocals.

BIFOCAL DISPENSING

Bifocal segments must be positioned so that the distance and near positions of the lens provide adequate fields of view for distance and near vision respectively. The fitting position of the bifocal segments should be decided according to the purpose for which they are to be worn. However, it is necessary to consider the positioning of segments in vertical and horizontal meridians. So while dispensing bifocal lenses three factors as shown in **Flowchart 10.5** must be considered:

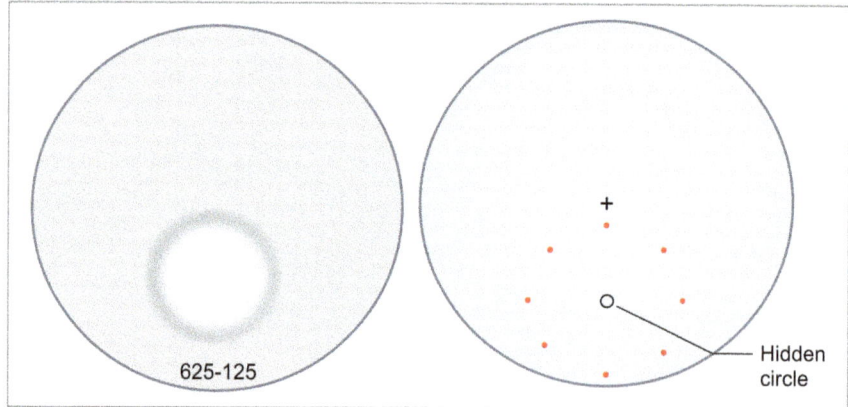

Fig. 10.23: Invisible bifocal-round shape

Flowchart 10. 5: Factors to consider while dispensing bifocal Lenses

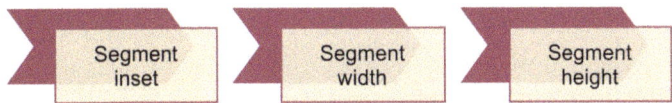

Segment Inset

Segment inset is specified as the difference between the subjects distance PD and near PD. In the normal range of PDs, the near PD for a reading distance of 40cms is 4mm less than the distance PD. Segment inset, therefore, is usually specified as 2mm for each lens. There are two reasons for insetting bifocal segment – to ensure that the subject's line of sight will go through the segment at its optical center and to ensure that the reading fields for the two segments will coincide with one another.

Segment Width

Different segment widths are usually available for straight top shaped segments in 22, 25, 28 and 35 mm widths. Some manufacturers also provide this option in round shaped segments. E-style bifocal encompasses the full width of the lens, so it is obvious not to specify segment width when this lens is prescribed. Given a choice wider segment widths are preferred.

Segment Height

In the vertical meridian, bifocal lenses prescribed for general purpose use are usually mounted before the eyes so that the segment top is tangential to the lower edge of the iris **(Fig. 10.24A)**. In most cases the position of the lower edge of the iris also corresponds with the line of the lower eyelid when the head is held in the primary position. This is usually normal for great majority of bifocal wearers and is certainly the safest position for the segment top in case of first time wearers. However, if the bifocal prescribed is mainly for near vision, then the segment top might be fitted little higher, say, midway between the lower edge of the iris and the lower edge of the pupil **(Fig. 10.24B)**. If the lenses have been prescribed for some vocational purpose and are to be designed for only occasional near vision use, then the segment top might be fitted 2-3 mm lower than the normal **(Fig. 10.24C)**.

These suggested positions of the segment top assume that the head is held in the subjects primary position with the eyes viewing a distant object. But if a person who habitually holds his head high will need a lower segment height than a person who slouches a bit and keeps his head downward. A tall person who habitually keeps his head down may need a little higher segment top whereas a short height person who has to keep his head up may prefer a little down segment top. Past wearing habit of the subject should also be given

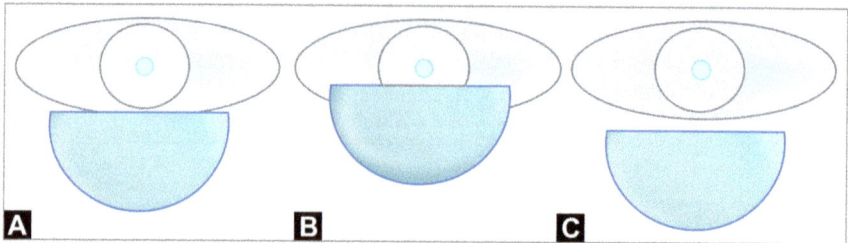

Figs. 10.24A to C: Placement of near segment height at different position

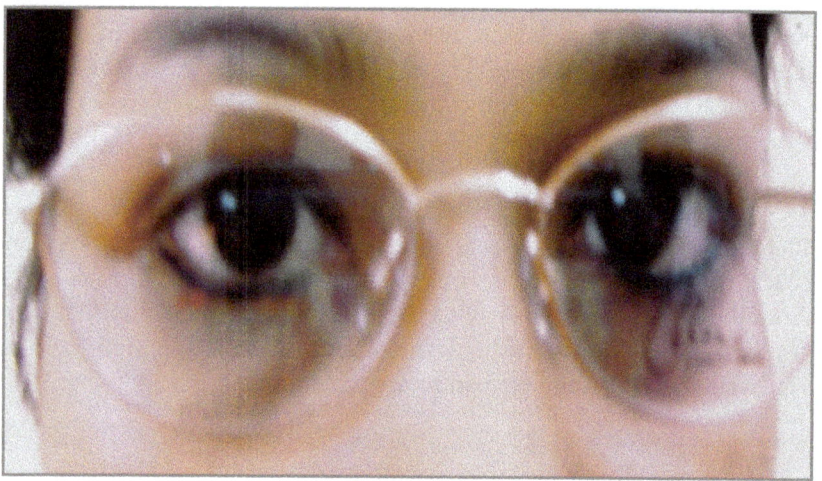

Fig. 10.25: Adjusted frame on wearer's face

importance while positioning the segment top. If a wearer is used to wearing bifocal segment up, fitting a lower segment in the new spectacle will create trouble for him to adjust immediately.

Various kinds of dispensing aids have been proposed from time to time to assist in the fitting of bifocal lenses, but most practitioners obtain excellent and consistent results by simply measuring the segment height with a millimeter ruler. Ideally the segment height should be converted into a segment top position in relation to the horizontal center line of the frame. A typical routine procedure for taking the measurement is:

- Choose the final frame and adjust it to fit the subject correctly with appropriate pantoscopic angle, front bow and nose pads fitting **(Fig. 10.25)**.
- If the frame is without demonstration lens, attach a vertical strip of transparent adhesive tape to each eye of the frame to enable reference points to be marked **(Fig. 10.26)**.
- Replace the frame on the subjects face and direct the subject to look straight into your eyes. If necessary, adjust the height of your chair so that your eyes are on exactly the same level as those of the subject **(Fig. 10.27)**.

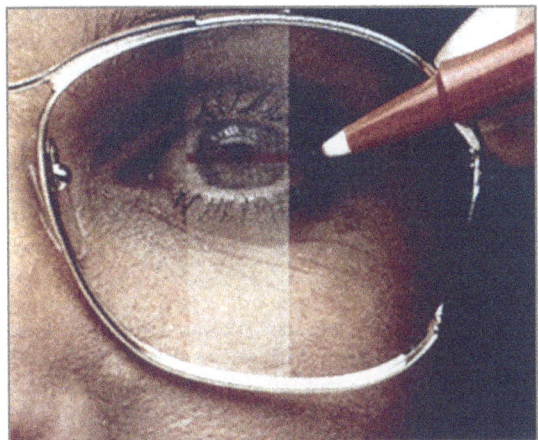

Fig. 10.26: Tap on frame eye wire

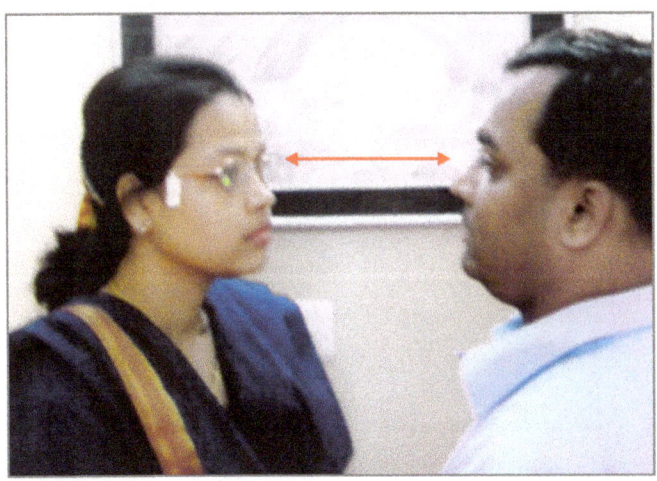

Fig. 10.27: Patient and practitioner standing opposite to each other at same height

- Direct the subject to look straight into your open left eyes and using a fine tip marking pen, place dots at the same height as the lower edge of the subject's right iris. This point often coincides with the line of the lower lid. Similarly, without moving his head, place a second mark in front of the subjects left lower iris margin **(Fig. 10.28)**.
- Remove the frame and put the frame face down with dots coinciding with a straight line. Draw a straight line from one dot to another **(Fig. 10.29)**.
- Put back the frame on the face and verify **(Fig. 10.30)**.
- The position of the segment top is usually specified in millimeter from the marked straight line to the lower eye wire of the frame where the bevel of the lens will fit into the groove **(Fig. 10.31)**.

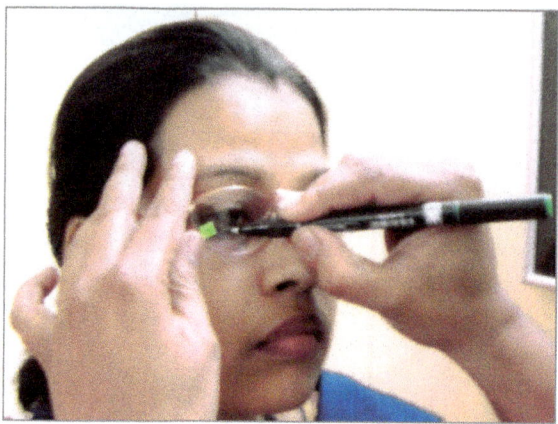

Fig. 10.28: Marking on lens insert with reference to lower lid

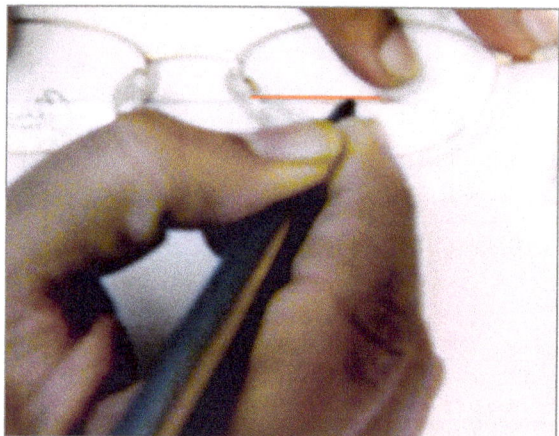

Fig. 10.29: Marking straight line on lens insert

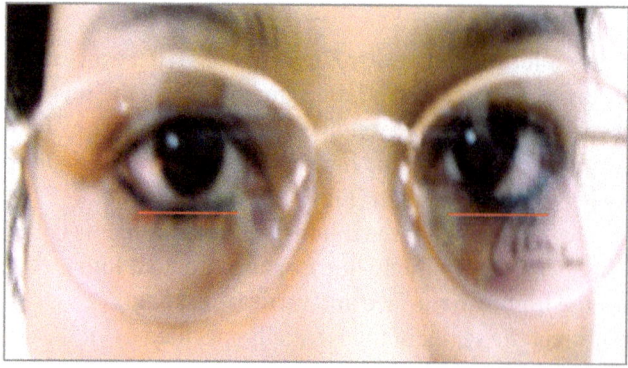

Fig. 10.30: Reference line marked in line with the edge of lower lid

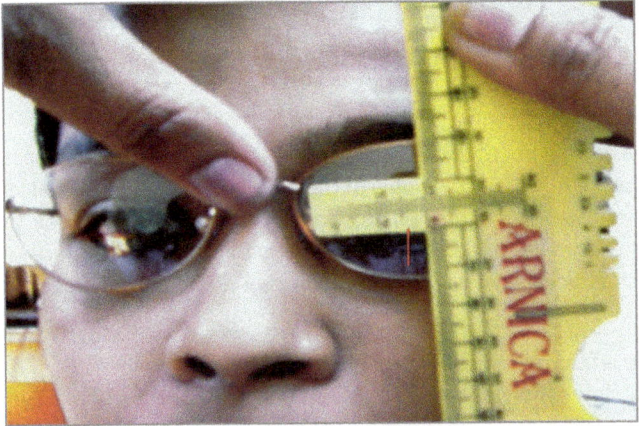

Fig. 10.31: Using scale to measure vertical height from lower rim

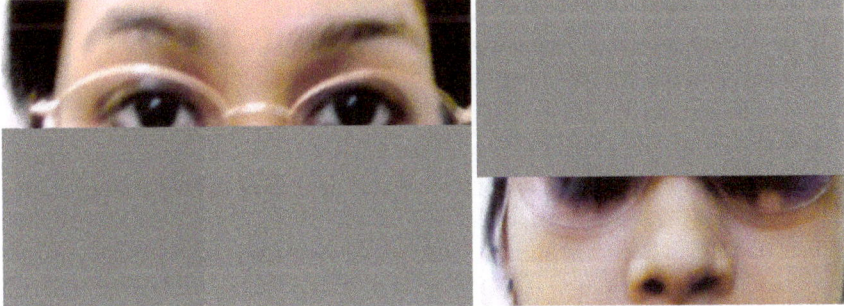

Fig. 10.32: Verifying for segment height

VERIFICATION OF SEGMENT HEIGHT

Subjective determination is the most accurate means of determining the segment height and of assuring the wearer that the bifocal segment will be positioned properly **(Fig. 10.32)**.

- Ask the subject to stand and look straight ahead.
- A card is held over the lower half of the frame with its upper border coinciding with the proposed segment position.
- The subject should be able to see the floor over the top of the card at a distance of 15 feet.
- Now ask the subject to look down at the reading material. The card is held over the upper portion of the frame with its lower border at the level of the proposed bifocal segment.
- The reading material should be visible without major readjustments of the subject's posture or reading material.

Multiple Choice Questions (MCQs)

1. Which of the following is not *true* about bifocal lenses?
    a. The near segment of the bifocal lenses is usually inferior and nasally shifted.
    b. Prisms cannot be made only in the near portion of the bifocal lens.
    c. When the line of gaze passes from distance to near to look through the near segment of the lens, there is a possibility of image jump.
    d. Fused bifocal involves the use of lenses with different refractive indices.

2. The amount of reading addition in fused bifocal lenses depends upon…..
    a. The refractive indices of two glass materials
    b. The depression curve
    c. The curve worked on the segment side of the lens
    d. All of the above

3. Which of the following cannot work to minimize the effect of image jump in bifocal lenses?
    a. Adding base up prism to the reading portion of the lens
    b. Moving the optical center of the lens near the junction of the two portions
    c. Applying pantoscopic tilt to the spectacle frame
    d. Using E-style bifocal lenses

4. Which of the following type of bifocal lens does not produce image jump?
    a. Round shaped bifocal lens
    b. D-shaped bifocal lens
    c. E-style bifocal lens
    d. None of the above

Answers

1. b   2. d   3. c   4. c

Chapter 11

Progressive Addition Lenses

The concept of progressive addition lens has been around since 1907 when the first patent on progressive power lens was published by Owen Ave. The early progressive lenses were rather crude in design. Varilux 1 was introduced by Essilor in France in the year 1959 and since then progressive addition lens have gained worldwide acceptance as the most performing ophthalmic lens for the correction of presbyopia because they provide comfortable vision at all distances. They have successfully and advantageously replaced single vision and bifocal lenses. Growing popularity of progressive addition lenses has stimulated the search for advances in design and manufacturing technology of the progressive lenses. This has enabled progressive addition lenses to develop from the early "hard" designs requiring extended patient adaptation time to current "state of the art" softer asymmetric design to the individually customized progressive lenses. Today over 150 progressive addition lens designs are in the market.

Progressive addition lenses (**Fig. 11.1**) are one piece lenses that vary gradually in surface curvature from a minimum value in the upper distance portion to a maximum value in the lower near portion. Unlike bifocal or trifocal

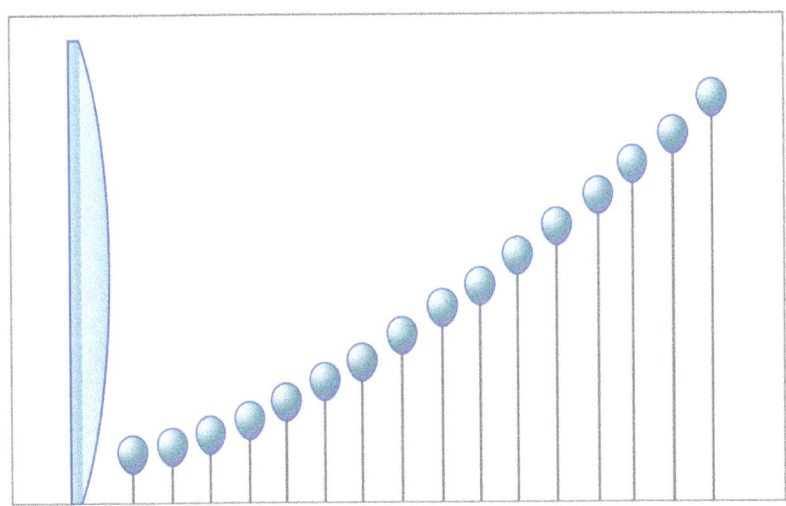

Fig. 11.1: Progressive addition lens

lenses, progressive lenses ensure that the presbyopic spectacle wearer finds the right dioptric power for every distance, guaranteeing smooth and uninterrupted vision without any visible line of demarcation. The power increase is achieved by constantly decreasing the radii of curvature in the vertical and horizontal directions. **Figure 11.2** demonstrates the gradual increase in curvature and surface power towards the lower, near portion of the lens.

In the most used zones of vision, virtually aberration-free vision is possible, as here the radii of curvature are almost identical in the vertical and horizontal directions.

A typical, general-purpose progressive lens will have three district zones of vision as shown in **Figure 11.3**.

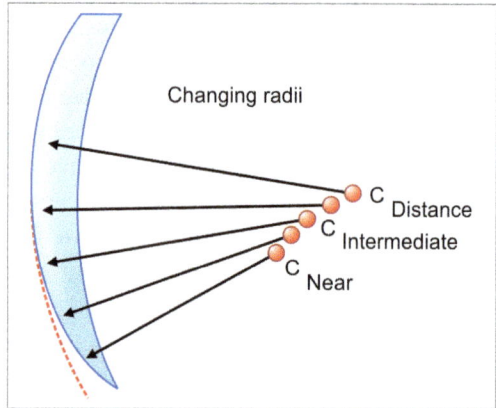

Fig. 11.2: Cross-sectional view of progressive addition lens surface. The shorter radius of curvature in near portion provides a stronger surface power than the longer radius of curvature in the distance portion

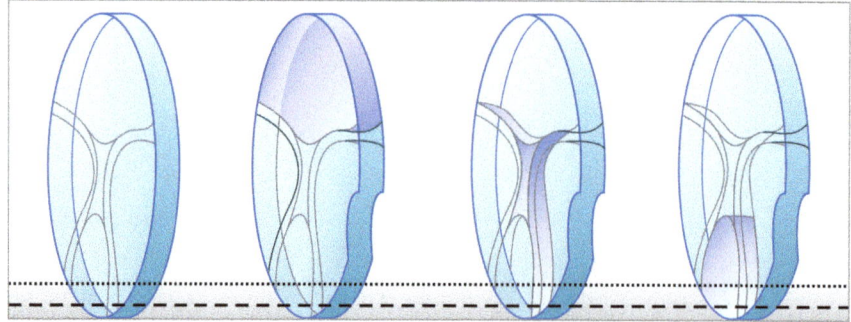

Fig. 11.3: Distance, intermediate and near zones of a typical progressive lens

DISTANCE

Distance viewing zone is defined by the stable distance power in the upper portion of the lens. It represents the width of the clear distance vision with the eye in straight ahead position. Distance reference point, fitting cross, prism reference point all lie within distance viewing zone.

NEAR

Near vision zone is defined by the stable spherical near addition into the lower part of the lens. It represents the width of the clear near vision with the eye in down gaze position. Near reference point lies within this zone on umbilic where the full target addition is achieved.

INTERMEDIATE

A corridor in the central portion of the lens connects above two zones, which increase progressively in plus power from the distance to near. This zone is also known as "progressive zone". It provides intermediate or mid range viewing zone. The width and utility of the intermediate distance viewing zone varies depending upon the wearer's tolerance to blur.

These three zones of vision blend together seamlessly, providing the wearer with a continuous depth of field from near to far (**Fig. 11.4**).

BASIC DESIGN DIFFERENCE BETWEEN PROGRESSIVE, SINGLE VISION, BIFOCAL AND TRIFOCAL LENSES

A single vision reading lens consists of a single sphere of appropriate radius providing correction for near vision only. Distance vision through the lens is blurred and there is no specific correction for the intermediate vision. (**Fig. 11.5**).

They provide larger field of view for the reading and they are readily available at low cost. But they are inconvenient to use as they correct only one particular distance at a time.

Bifocal, trifocal and progressive lens designs combine areas of correction for both distance and near vision in a single lens and link them in different ways:

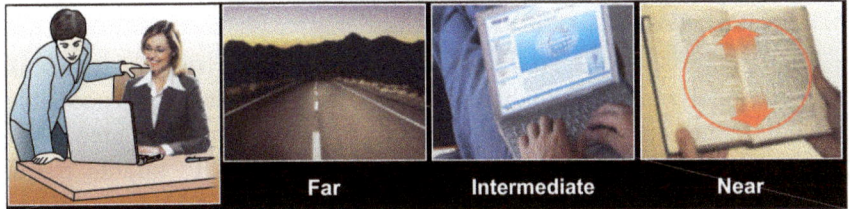

Fig. 11.4: Typical progressive lens

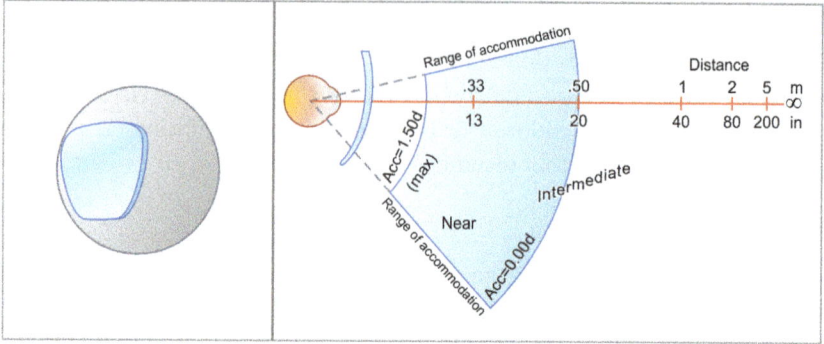

Fig. 11.5: Basic design principle of single vision lens

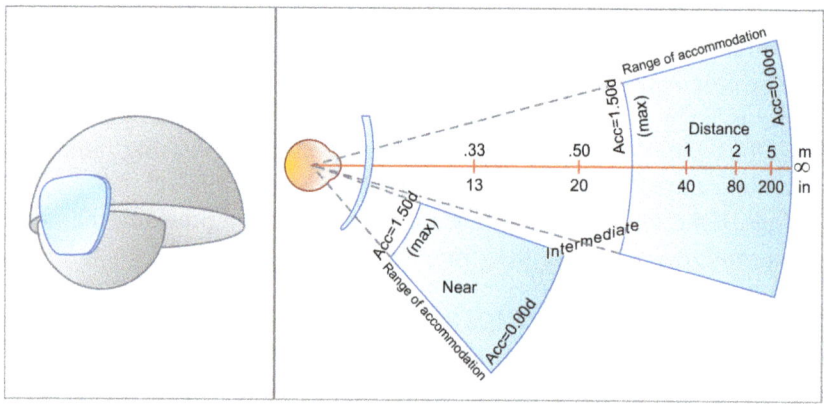

Fig. 11.6: Design principle of bifocal lens

In a bifocal lens, a distance vision sphere is placed above a near vision sphere and is linked by a single "step" creating a visible segment line. They offer convenience of distance and near in the same spectacle and are available at lower cost. But they are unappealing cosmetically as there is a visible demarcation between zones. Intermediate is blurred and the subject have prismatic image jump **(Fig. 11.6)**.

In a trifocal lens, a third sphere is added between the distance and near vision sphere to produce an intermediate power. This gives rise to two segment lines on the lens surface **(Fig. 11.7)**.

In a progressive lens, an uninterrupted series of horizontal curves link distance vision zone, intermediate vision zone and near vision with no visible separation. Lens power increases smoothly from distance vision area at the top of the lens, through an intermediate vision area in the middle, to the near vision area at the bottom of the lens. They provide convenience of use with no prismatic image jump. The subject feels confidence in negotiating

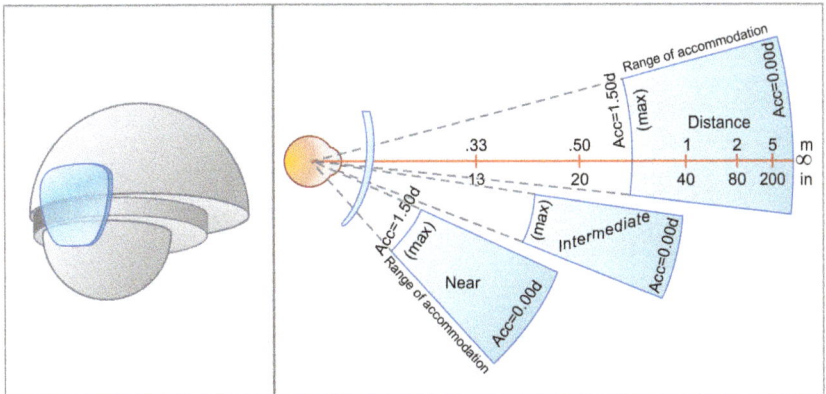

Fig. 11.7: Trifocal lens design principle

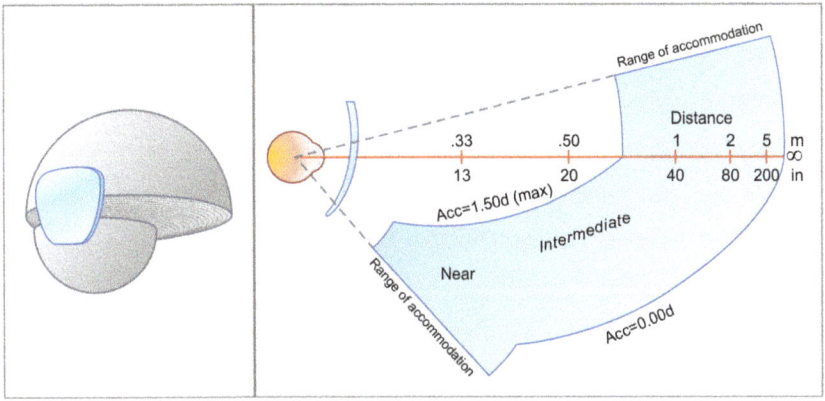

Fig.11.8: Progressive lens design principle

stairs; gutters, etc. Progressive addition lenses are under constant research and development, providing us a newer and better design to adapt faster **(Fig. 11.8)**.

ADVANTAGES OF PROGRESSIVE ADDITION LENSES

Most eyewear professionals are aware of the product benefits offered by the optical features of a progressive addition lens:

No Visible Segments

No line of demarcation provides more cosmetically appealing lenses with continuous vision, free from visually distracting borders. The lens looks like a single vision lens **(Fig. 11.9)**.

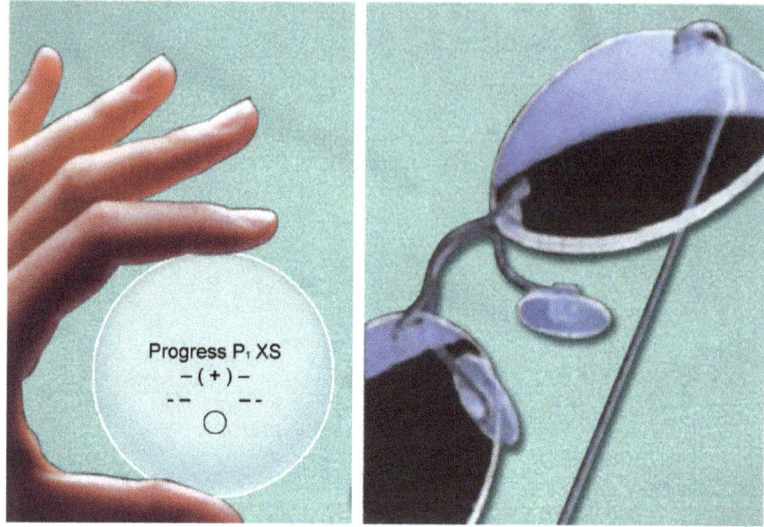

Fig. 11.9: No line progressive lens

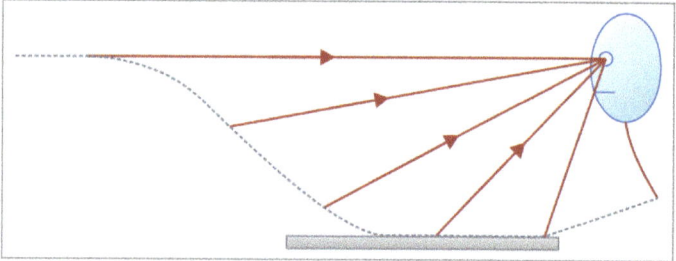

Fig. 11.10: Progressive lens provides clear vision from far to near

Continuous Field of Clear Vision

Progressive addition lens offers a greater visual flexibility with uninterrupted clear vision from distance to near. Single vision lenses are designed either for distance vision or for near vision or it may also be designed for occupational purpose, providing clear vision at a specific distance only, while the abrupt change of power in a bifocal creates completely divided fields for distance and near vision with no specific correction for intermediate vision. At virtually every point in the progressive lens, the eye finds the power in the perfect agreement with the distance at which it is focusing **(Fig. 11.10)**.

Comfortable Intermediate Vision

The progressive zone of the progressive addition lens gives rise to an area, which provides the clear vision for the intermediate correction **(Fig. 11.11)**. Only in the early stage of presbyopia, can single vision and bifocal wearer

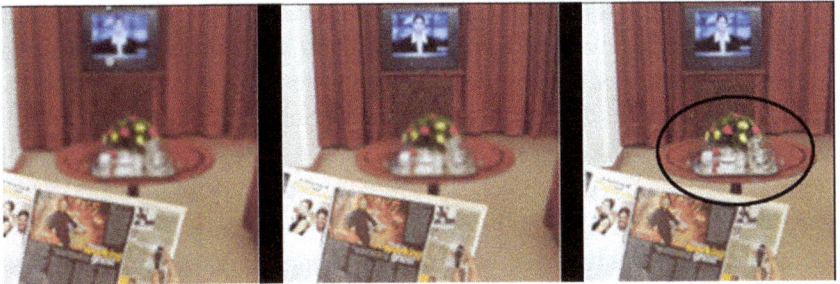

Fig. 11.11: Extreme right picture shows clear intermediate vision through progressive lens

enjoy clear intermediate vision, as they can still accommodate and adjust their head position. But for higher additions, progressive addition lens continues to offer clear vision at intermediate distance also. Trifocal lens, despite their clear intermediate field of vision, is not ideal, as the wearer must cope with the image jump at the two segment lenses.

Continuous Support to the Eyes Accommodation

In a single vision-reading lens, the eyes accommodation is supported for near vision only. In a bifocal lens, the eyes accommodation experiences abrupt changes when the gaze shifts from distance to near vision across the segment lines, because the wearer must constantly choose between distance and near vision power and switch from maximum to minimum amplitude of accommodation. For example, consider an eye focusing through a bifocal lens at an object moving towards it from a reasonable distance. The eye first uses the distance power, accommodating to its maximum amplitude to focus as the object is drawn within arm's length. The eye then switches to the near segment where it must totally relax its accommodation for intermediate viewing, before again increasing to its maximum amplitude of accommodation as the object is drawn closer. Thus, the eye varies its amplitude of accommodation twice from minimum to maximum. This adjustment in accommodation would occur only once with a progressive lens, just as it would with natural, non-presbyopic accommodation.

Continuous Perception of Space

Progressive lens also offers global perception of space in all direction, uninterrupted by any limitations or divisions. Changes of power are gradual and continuous in all directions with minimum distortion. Single vision lenses, if designed for only reading purpose, limits the spatial perception to the specific distance, while single vision lenses designed for distance vision do not allow perception of near field of vision. The two portions of bifocal lenses split and alter spatial relationship. Vertical and horizontal lines appear broken and image jump affects wearer's vision. A progressive addition lens is designed not only to provide clear and continuous vision at all distances but also to ensure natural and continuous perceptions of space in all directions. However, designing constraints distorts the spatial perception in extreme lateral gaze as shown in **Figure 11.12**.

■ PROGRESSIVE ADDITION LENS MARKINGS

All the progressive addition lenses contain important markings, which are used to identify lenses and to assist in their fitting and verification. The important markings are explained in **Figure 11.13**.

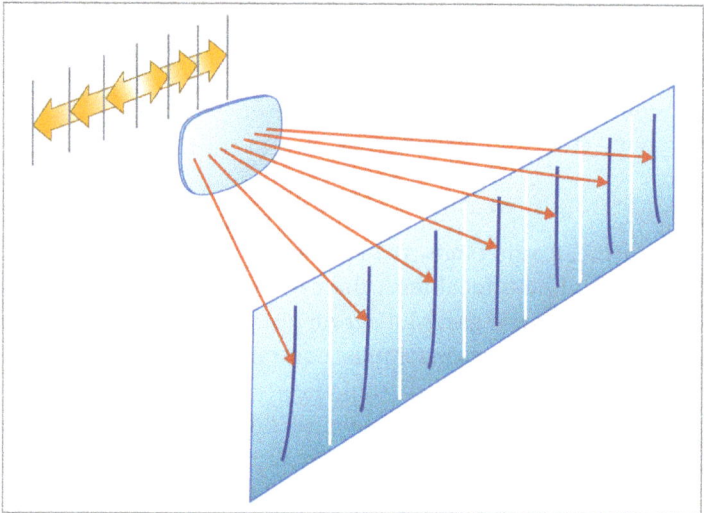

Fig. 11.12: Perception of form and movement through a progressive lens

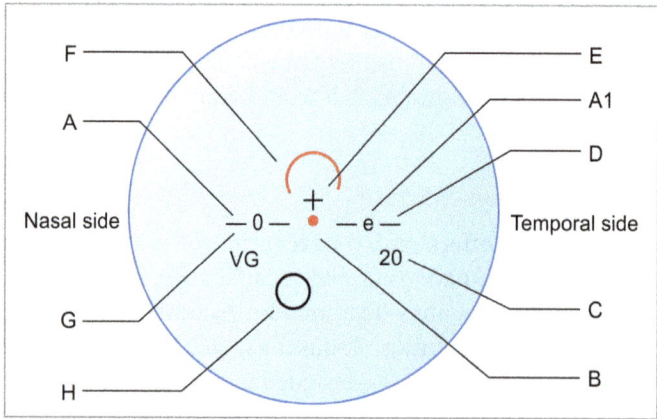

Fig. 11.13: Left eye progressive lens

A and A1: They are two hidden circles, which are permanently etched on the lens at 34 mm apart. When the ink marking is removed, they are made visible by fogging.
B: This point is the distance optical center (DOC) of the lens and is also known as prism reference point.
C: Hidden addition power situated at the temporal side and is made visible by fogging.
D: 0–180° axis line passing through the DOC.
E: Fitting cross lies above the DOC.
F: This is the distance power (DP) circle to check the exact distance power with the help of lensometer.
G: Hidden logo situated nasally and is made visible by fogging when the ink marking is removed.
H: 7 mm to 9 mm circle is the center of the near vision area and is inset by 2.5 mm.

PROGRESSIVE ADDITION LENS OPTICAL DESIGN

A typical progressive addition lens is designed to have several specific zones as shown in **Figure 11.14**:
- Distance viewing zone
- Near viewing zone
- Intermediate viewing zone
- Progressive corridor
- Blending region.

Each zone is seamlessly blended to ensure globally smooth surface that provides a gradual transition in curvature from the distance portion down to the near portion. This gradual blending of curvature means that the addition power is gradually changing across a large area of the lens. Unfortunately, the superior optics and line free nature of progressive addition lens does have a bit of a price to pay, i.e., the change in curvature results in an inevitable

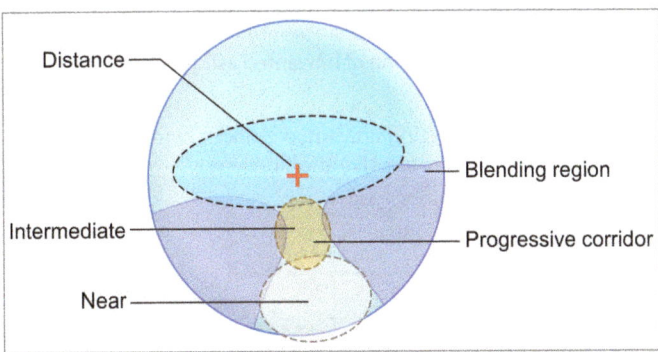

Fig. 11.14: Typical anatomy of progressive addition lens

consequence in the form of surface astigmatism at the temporal and nasal side. Surface astigmatism produces an unwanted astigmatic error or cylinder error that can blur vision and limit the wearers field of clear vision. Therefore, this astigmatic error essentially serves as a boundary for the various zones on the progressive lens surface as shown in **Figure 11.15**.

Unwanted cylinder which is the consequence of the lens design is influenced by 3 factors as shown by **Flowchart 11.1**.

Addition Power

The near addition is achieved by changing the curvature of the progressive addition lens along the umbilic from fitting cross position going down to the near reference point which causes astigmatism on either side of the umbilic line. The amount of astigmatism will be directly proportional to the add power of the lens. A +2.00 D addition, for example will generally produce twice as much cylinder error as +1.00 D addition.

Length of the Progressive Corridor

Shorter corridors produce more rapid power change and higher levels of astigmatism, but reduce the eye movement required to reach the near zone.

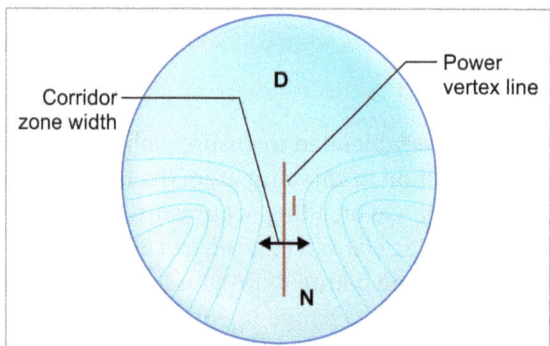

Fig. 11.15: The widths of the error-free distance, intermediate, and near largely depends upon the magnitude and distribution of unwanted astigmatism across lens designs

Flowchart 11.1: Factors affecting unwanted cylinder in the peripheral zones of progressive addition lens

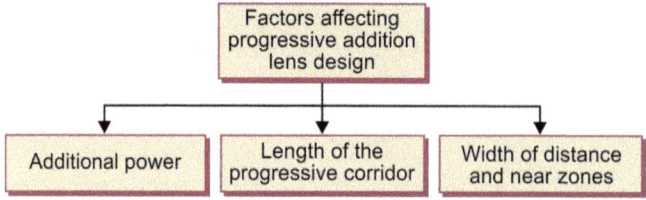

Larger corridors provide subtle power changes and lower levels of astigmatism, but increase the eye movement required to reach the near zone of the lens.

Width of Distance and Near Zone

Wider distance and near zones confine the astigmatism to smaller regions of the lens surface, which produces higher levels of astigmatism. However, wider zones do provide larger areas of clear vision. The location of the near zone, which is offset nasally to account for convergence in down gaze, is critical to wearer's comfort and its position varies between designs.

To understand how the length of the progressive corridor and the add power can affect the rate of change and magnitude of the astigmatic error, consider a progressive lens with a + 2.50 D addition, which has a 17 mm progressive corridor. This lens will have to change by 2.50 over a distance of 17 mm. This implies plus power represents an average change of roughly 2.50/17 = 0.15 D per millimeter. Therefore, the power of a progressive lens changes more rapidly down the progressive corridor as the addition power increases or the length of the corridor decreases. A well designed progressive lens will reduce the amount of astigmatic error to its mathematical limits for a given design.

During the design and optimization process, various parameters are adjusted to control and manipulate the distribution and magnitude of this astigmatic error across the progressive lens surface. The width of the near and distance zones, and the length of the progressive corridor are the chief parameters that are altered. The overall power profile of a progressive addition lens as shown in **Figure 11.16** is characterized by appropriate power progression along the vertical direction by associating the shape of the power progression to the orientation of reading material linked to the natural convergence of eye movement during the near vision.

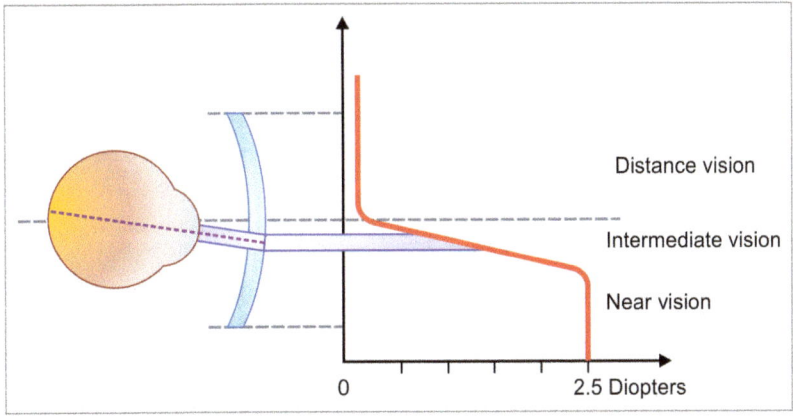

Fig. 11.16: Power profile for a progressive lens

The magnitude, distribution and the rate of change of this astigmatism error are all performance factors that can affect the wearers acceptance of the lens. The amount and distribution of cylinder at the lens peripheral portion determines the field of view, while the rate of change and orientation of cylinder primarily influence adaptation time. A steeper distribution concentrates the change in cylinder over a smaller distance and provides wider distance and near zones free of aberration.

> Astigmatic aberration is generally perceived as distortion or blur while prismatic aberration is perceived as "swim" or "waviness" with head movement.

MINKWITZ RULE

Minkwitz theorem shows how corridor width of the progressive addition lenses is determined with respect to the variation in near addition of the lens. Minkwitz suggested three important points:
1. Any change in power curve along umbilic gives rise to surface astigmatism perpendicular to it. Astigmatism starts immediately beside the center line.
2. Rate of change in surface astigmatism is twice the rate of power change along the umbilic.
3. Maximum surface astigmatism around the umbilic is proportional to the add power.

Mathematically, Minkwitz Rule can be described as:
$$x = AST * h/2A$$
where,
- AST is the amount of astigmatism
- A is the full near addition
- h is the progression depth of the near addition
- x is the distance from the umbilic line to the amount of astigmatism.

> The width of progressive corridor means defining the limits of unwanted surface astigmatism that surrounds the center line.

PROGRESSIVE ADDITION LENS DESIGNS

Broadly, the progressive addition lens design can be categorized into three groups as shown in **Figure 11.17**.

Mono Design and Multidesign

In case of mono design progressive addition lens, a single design is used for all addition powers, i.e. the position for the near vision does not change with the change in near addition power causing difficulties while viewing near objects as the wearer holds reading material closer to him with the increase in his near addition power. Hence, it can never offer optimum comfort to both emerging presbyopes and matured presbyopes, as their needs are different.

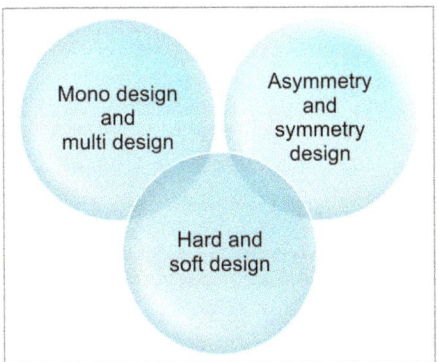

Fig. 11.17: Progressive addition lens design

In multidesign the position for near vision changes with the addition power change, i.e., the near area goes up with the increase in the addition. All the twelve additions from 0.75 D to 3.50 D have been studied separately to define the ideal design for each stage of presbyopes.

Asymmetry and Symmetry Design (Fig. 11.18)

In case of symmetrical progressive addition lens design, the right and the left lenses are identical. To achieve the desired inset for the near zone, they are simply rotated by an equal and opposite amount in the two lenses, i.e., 10° anti-clockwise in the right lens and clockwise in the left lens. The principal drawback of this design is the disruption of binocular vision as the wearer gazes laterally across the lens, since the astigmatism differed between the nasal and temporal sides of the distance zone.

Asymmetric progressive addition lens design incorporates a nasal offset of the near zone and has separate design for right and left lens. So, there is no need of lens rotation in this case. This results in same peripheral optical characteristics and better adaptation, improved binocular vision, more visual comfort and better convergence.

Hard and Soft Design (Fig. 11.19)

A harder progressive addition lens design concentrates the astigmatic error into smaller areas of the lens surface, thereby expanding the areas of perfectly clear vision at the expense of higher levels of blur and distortion. Consequently, harder progressive addition lens generally exhibits four characteristics when compared to softer designs:
- Wider distance zones
- Wider near zones
- More narrow and shorter progressive corridors
- More rapidly increasing levels of astigmatic error

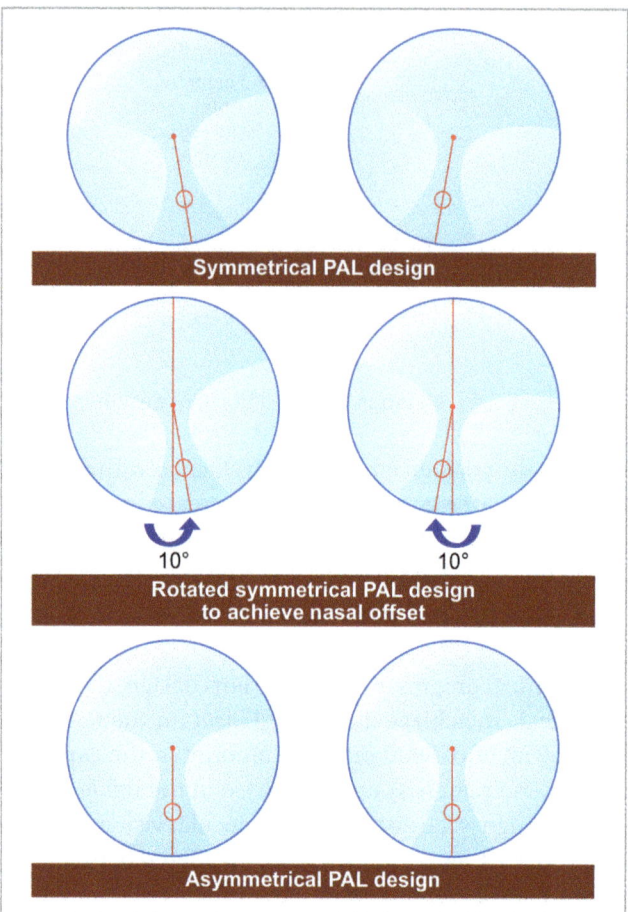

Fig. 11.18: Symmetrical and asymmetrical progressive addition lens design

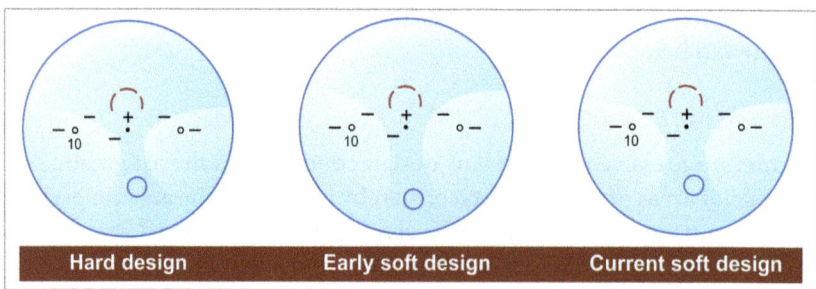

Fig. 11.19: Progressive addition lens designs with different varying concentration of cylinder error

A softer progressive addition lens design spreads the astigmatic error across larger areas of the surface, thereby reducing the overall magnitude of blur at the expense of narrowing the zones of perfectly clear vision. The astigmatic error may even encroach well into the distance zone. Consequently softer progressive addition lens generally exhibits four characteristics when compared to harder designs:
- Narrower distance zones
- Narrower near zones
- Longer and wider progressive corridors
- More slowly increasing levels of astigmatic error.

In general, harder progressive addition lens designs will provide wider fields of view, and will require less head and eye movement, at the expense of more swim and blur. Softer progressive addition lens designs provide reduced levels of astigmatism and swim while limiting the size of the zones of clear vision and requiring more head and eye movement.

However, modern progressive addition lenses are seldom absolutely "hard" or absolutely "soft". Unfortunately such terms do not accurately describe modern lenses. Many of the recent progressive addition lens design incorporates the best balance of these two design philosophies to show following characteristics:
- Larger effective distance and near zones
- Peripheral aberrations are well controlled to enable the wearer to adapt easily.
- Combination of hard and soft design.

Recently, Sola optical introduced another concept, i.e. design by prescription the use of different distance designs for different distance refractive errors. For example, the design employed for the 7.25 base curves varies slightly from the design employed for the 5.25 base.

■ OPTICAL DESCRIPTION OF PROGRESSIVE ADDITION LENS

Manufacturers have made various attempts to represent the size and location of the optical zones and peripheral aberrations of the progressive lens using several approaches. Graphically, four approaches have been used commonly to represent the progressive lens design as shown by **Flowchart 11.2** that

Flowchart 11.2: Methods to represent progressive addition lens (PAL) design

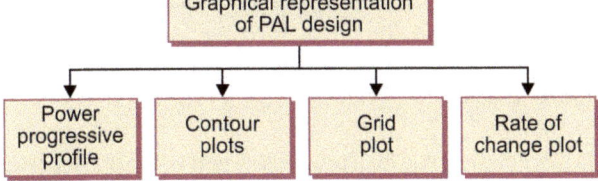

represent difference in overall distribution of power and astigmatism across the lens surface, indicating different design which may be used to establish the baseline for selecting an ideal progressive lens design for a patient based upon his visual need.

Power Progressive Profile

The primary function of a progressive addition lens is to restore near and intermediate vision while maintaining clear distance vision. While distance power and the near vision power in any given lens are fixed parameters, the lens design must define the progression of power change from one to the other. Physiological considerations favor a high location of the near vision zone; however, a short abrupt power progression from distance zone to near zone will usually create the rapidly varying aberrations in the lens periphery that cause discomfort. The great challenge for the designer is to manage both the length of the power progression and the rate of power change in order to create comfortable exploration of distance, intermediate and near visual fields without excessive, and tiring vertical head movements and ocular effort. The rate at which the power increases over the progressive zone is governed by the power law for the design. The power law may be linear as assumed in **Figure 11.20** or it may be more complex to provide a greater or less increase in power at the start of the progression as assumed in the **Figure 11.21**.

The curve so drawn represents the power progression of the lens along its meridional line from distance to near vision. The power progression is the result of a continuous shortening of the radius of curvature of the front surface.

Contour Plots

The contour plot is the most common method used to represent progressive addition lens designs. It describes the surface power of the front surface of the lens and identifies zones of constant surface power indicated by contour

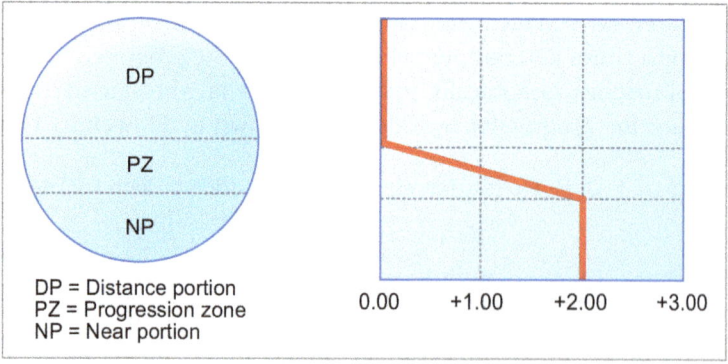

Fig. 11.20: Power profile for a progressive lens with a linear power law

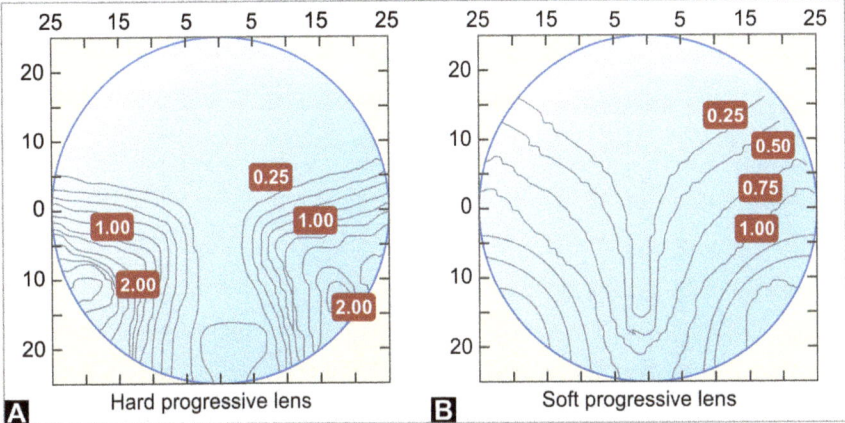

Fig. 11.21: Comparison of isocylinder lines for hard and soft design of power, plano add + 2.00 D

lines. Contour Plots also attempt to show the size of the distance, intermediate and near zones as well as the extent and gradient of peripheral aberrations. There are two types of contour plots:
1. Isosphere contour plots
2. Isocylinder contour plots

Isosphere Contour Plots

This is a two dimensional map of the lens representing the distribution of spherical power across the lens. This form of graphical representation divides the lens along lines of equal dioptric values. Each contour line/shade represents an increasing level of power at given interval. The value of this line/shade is chosen arbitrarily, usually at the increments of 0.25 D or 0.50 D to 1.00 D. Between two consecutive lines, sphere value varies by a relatively constant rate. **Figure 11.22** shows isosphere contour plot of a progressive addition lens. In addition to describing sphere distribution the lens designer may communicate information about the location and size of the near vision zone using an isosphere contour plot.

Isocylinder Contour Plots

Isocylinder contour plots are two-dimensional map that divides the lens design into ranges of cylinder levels through out the lens. Most of the time isocylinder plot is misused by the lens designer in the promotion of their progressive addition lenses. It is routinely misapplied by some lens marketer seeking to establish competitive claims such as "a larger reading zone" or "less unwanted astigmatism". Since induced cylinder is disturbing but unavoidable by progressive addition lens design process, it is legitimate for

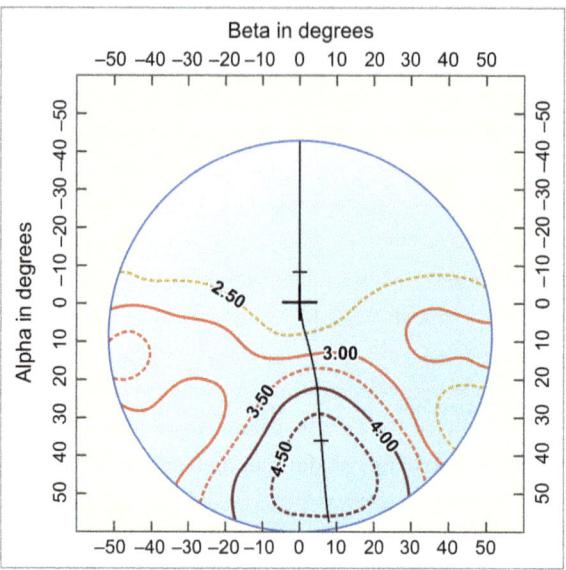

Fig. 11.22: Power contour plot of a PAL (+ 2.00 with a addition + 2.50 D)

the lens designers to map the location and degree of cylinder with each design interaction. "Soft" design have fewer zones of induced cylinder, represented by fewer lines on the isocylinder contour plots, located further apart than in "hard" design. Hard designs, on the other hand, have a greater number of lines located closer together. To the untrained observer, the hard design may appear superior because of the longer areas free of induced cylinder. However, clinical experience has shown that wearers perceive soft design as more comfortable in dynamic and peripheral vision as they do not have a high concentration of cylinder in areas critical to peripheral and dynamic vision, as in the case with hard designs **(Fig. 11.23)**.

Lens designers also use isocylinder contour plots to depict the presence or absence of asymmetry in the progressive addition lens design by comparing the nasal and temporal aspects on either side of the oblique path of power progression. An asymmetric design produces identical optical characteristics on both sides and thus, sphere power cylinder, and vertical prism are almost identical for both eyes in any direction of gaze, promoting binocularity and comfort. A symmetric design employs a single design that is rotated about 10 degrees in one direction to create a "right" lens and about 10 degrees in the opposite direction to create a left lens. In a hybrid of these two approaches, referred to as dissymmetric design, separate designs are used for right and left lenses. However, since the entire unwanted cylinder has been pushed from the temporal to the nasal side, different optical characteristics are present on either side of the lens.

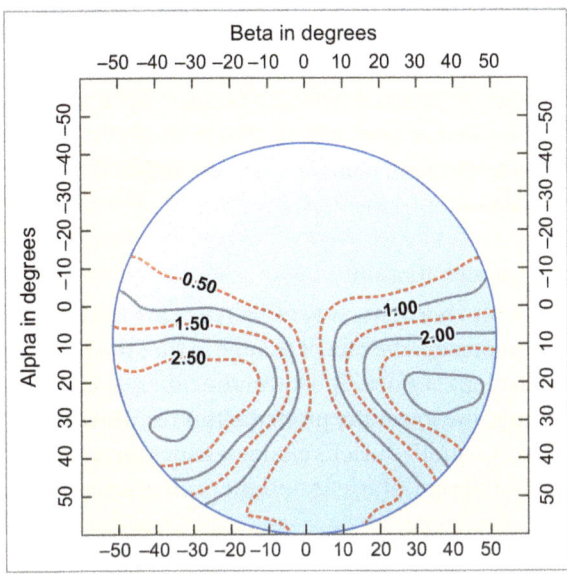

Fig. 11.23: Astigmatic contour plot of a PAL (+ 2.50 add)

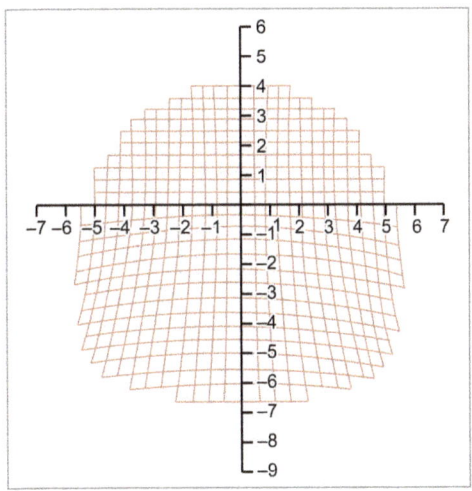

Fig. 11.24: Grid plot a PAL (+ 2.50D add)

Grid Plot (Fig. 11.24)

The grid highlights the distribution of the lens aberrations by showing how they alter a regular rectangular grid. The computational area of the lens surface is "discretized" by breaking regions of the surface up into square elements across a reference grid. Each intersection between these square elements represents a position on the lens surface, and contains some mathematical quantities that characterizes the surface at that point, including its local curvature.

Rate of Change Plot (Fig. 11.25)

Rate of change plots are the three dimensional graphical representation of the variation in the optical characteristics of progressive addition lenses, which plots vertically the value of a given optical characteristics at each point of the lens in relation to a reference plane. It may be used to show:
- Distribution of power
- Astigmatism
- Gradients of power variation

Rate of change plot is a better way to visualize the softness or hardness of a lens design. They represent the rate of change in the sphere value between two given points on the lens surface. The lower the difference in the sphere power between two points, the lower the plotted altitudes. Thus, three-dimensional plots are more demonstrative of lens characteristics than contour plots. Flatter plots indicate softer design. The lens designer can manage the softness in one of the two ways.
1. By lengthening the progression.
2. By carefully controlling the rate of change of the optical characteristics between all points on the lens surface.

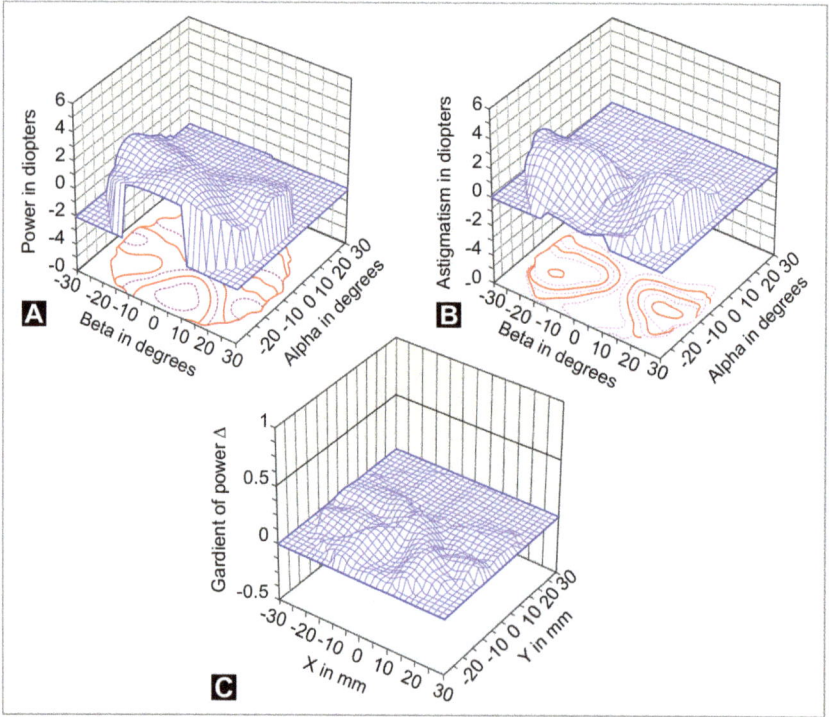

Figs. 11.25A to C: (A) 3D power plot of a PAL (+ 2.50 ADD); (B) 3D astigmatism plot of PAL (+ 2.50 ADD); (C) 3D power gradients plot of PAL (2.50 ADD)

Since the length of the power progression is not easily demonstrated on the rate of change plots, they give incomplete picture of the overall lens design. Otherwise this is a more demonstrative procedure.

The graphical representations are useful tools to communicate the geometrical features of PAL design to a trained observer. However, they do not really correlate with wearer's acceptance, as this is dependent on the sum total of many different factors—astigmatic error, the power rise, prismatic effects, distortions, the required dioptric power, cent ration, the frame fit, vertex distance and the subjective impression of the wearer. So the success of a progressive addition lens design should be judged on extensive wearing trials rather than studying as these plots.

DESIGNING PROGRESSIVE ADDITION LENS

A progressive addition lens is designed not only to provide a presbyope—an ability to see clearly at all distances but also to respect all the physiological visual functions like foveal vision, extra foveal vision, binocular vision, etc. The foveal area of the retina permits sharp vision at any distance within a small field which follows the eyes rotation which is usually within 30° angle.

Within this end the lens areas used for foveal vision must provide for perfect retinal images. The wearers natural body and head positions determine the vertical rotation of the eye for near and distance vision, and therefore the optimal length of the lens power progression. The co-ordination of the body, head and eye movements in relation to the objects location in the vision field defines the power value needed at each point of the progression. The horizontal eye and head movements determine the field of gaze and defines the width of the lens zone used for foveal vision. And to maximize wearers visual acuity in the lens central area, the unwanted induced cylinder of the progressive lens must be kept to a minimum and be pushed to the periphery of the lens.

Although, extra-foveal vision do not provide sharp vision but the wearer do locate the object in space, perceive their forms and detect their movements through extra-foveal vision. The prismatic distribution on the progressive addition lens surface and its magnitude introduces slight deformation of horizontal and vertical lines, thus altering the wearers visual comfort. The whole of the retina is almost homogeneously sensitive to motion. The variation of prismatic effects plays a role in the wearer's comfort where it must be slow and smooth across the whole lens to ensure comfortable dynamic vision **(Fig. 11.26)**.

Binocular vision refers to the simultaneous perception of the two eyes **(Fig. 11.27)**. For perfect fusion, the image produced by the right and left lenses must be formed as corresponding retinal points and display similar optical properties. The eyes naturally converge when the wearers gaze is lowered for

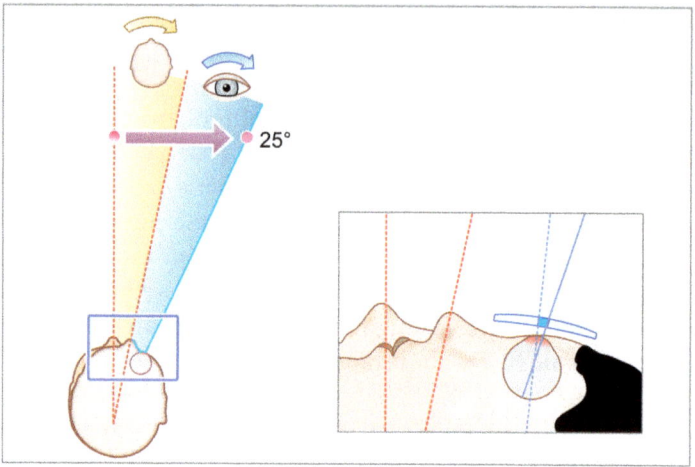

Fig. 11.26: Horizontal eye/head movement coordination and width of field

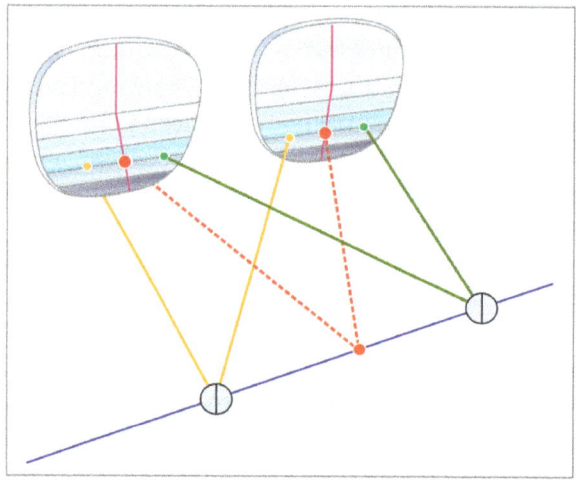

Fig. 11.27: Binocular vision with progressive lenses

near vision. The power progression must be positioned in the lens in such a manner that it follows the eyes path of convergence downwards in the nasal direction. Both right and left lenses must offer approximately equal vertical prism on each side of the progression path. The retinal images formed in both eyes must be similar in all directions of gaze. For that purpose, the power and astigmatism encountered on corresponding points of right and left lenses must be approximately equal.

In designing the following zones of the progressive addition lens, the lens designer works towards respecting these physiological functions:

Vertical Location of the Near Vision Area

Higher position of near vision area relieves strain to extra ocular muscles and eases binocular function with downward gaze. But a shorter progression usually results in rapidly varying peripheral aberrations. A good compromise consists in locating the usable near vision at a downward gaze position of about 25°.

Power Progression Profile

A suitable power progression along the meridional line enables the wearer to explore the object field without tiresome vertical head movements. This is achieved by associating the shape of the power progression to the orientation of the vertical horopter linked to the natural tilting of reading material **(Fig. 11.28)**.

Horizontal (Lateral) Location of the Near Vision Area

Once the power profile has been defined, its lateral positioning on the lens must be adapted to the natural convergence of the eyes and the value of the addition. With the advanced presbyopia, the reading distance becomes closer, the meridional line, therefore, must be shifted nasally as the addition increases.

Besides, balancing of vertical prism between right and left lens is very important to respect retinal image fusion in binocular vision. This is achieved by an asymmetrical design of the progressive addition lens surface coupled with proper positioning of the meridional line. In the lens periphery, image quality constraints are less demanding, while the control of prismatic effects is of utmost importance for motion perception.

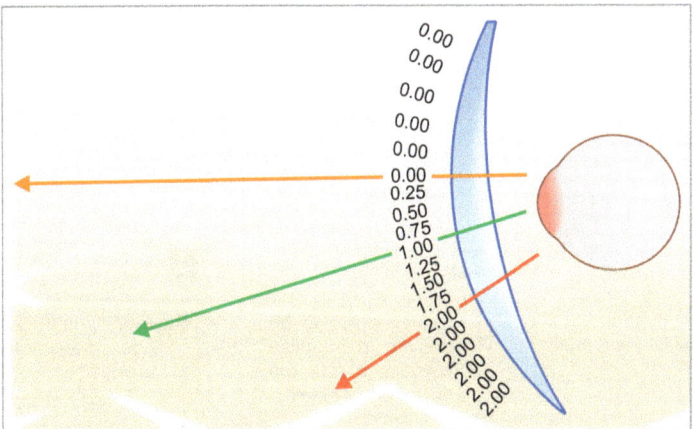

Fig. 11.28: Progression of power in relation to head posture and downward eye movement

All of the above optical requirements are introduced in the Merit function and are then integrated into the lens design optimization software. The merit function evaluates the numerous points of the lens and also overall performance of the lens by the weighted sum of the found merit function values and then the lens design is optimized. Numerous lens prototypes of each design are then produced and tested through rigorous clinical trials. Comparative lens evaluations are made after in depth analysis and patients comments, leading to a final selection of the progressive addition lens design.

■ PRISM THINNING (FIGS. 11.29A TO C)

The progressive addition lenses are designed by increasing the curvature of the progressive zone in the near vision area. As a result of this, the progressive addition lens is thinner at the bottom and thicker at the top. To produce a thinner lens, the lens surfaces generally use an "equithin" technique which consists of incorporating a vertical prism in order to reduce the thickness and weight of the lens in the back surface specification of the lens. Since the same amount of vertical prism is incorporated into both right and left lenses, there is relatively no prismatic effect for the wearer. This prism is often referred to as Yoked prism, as no net binocular prismatic effect is produced.

So prism thinning is the process of grinding prism into a progressive lens blank to reduce the thickness difference between the upper and the lower edges. Prism thinning typically involves grinding base down prism into the progressive lens. In addition to balancing the thickness difference between the top and the bottom of the lens blank, prism thinning also reduces the center thickness of the lens with plus and/or higher add powers. The overall reduction in thickness also makes the lens lighter in weight **(Fig. 11.30)**.

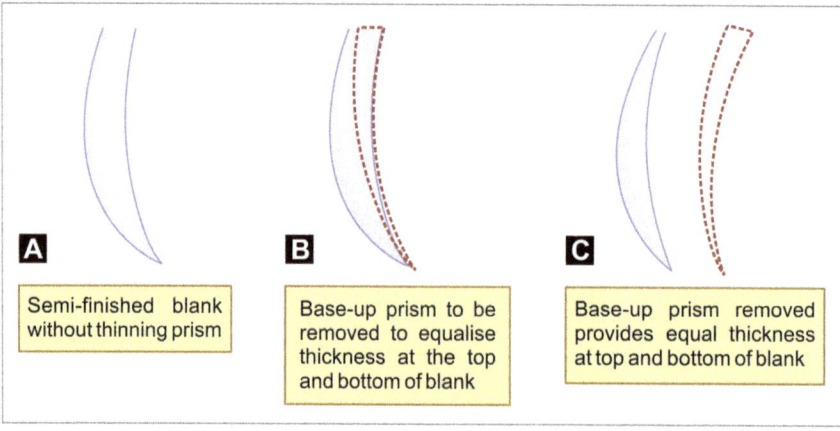

Figs. 11.29A to C: Thinning prism

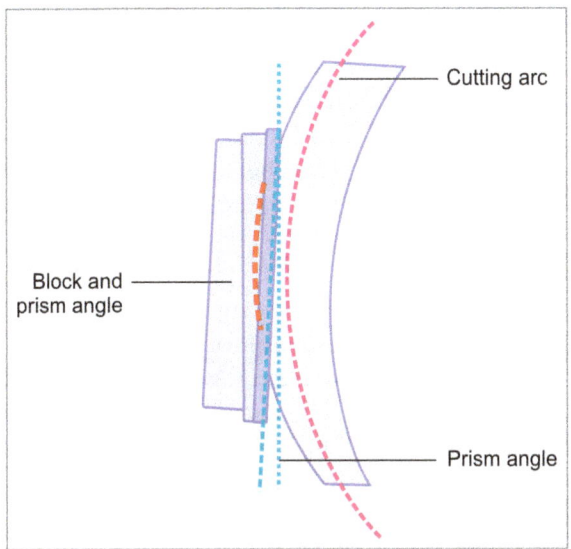

Fig. 11.30: Base down prism is ground into the lens blank using prism-ring (with its base positioned up) with conventional generators

Prism thinning is accomplished during the generating process by literally tilting the front surface of the lens on the chuck of conventional generator, using a base up positioned prism ring. When the back surface is ground normally, the surfaced lens is left with a prismatic effect at the center. Newer three axis generators produce this prismatic effect without the use of prism rings grinding the back curve with a tilt. The end result in either case is the reduction of unwanted thickness.

The amount of prism thinning used is roughly equal to the 2/3rd of the addition power. This is often recommended when the power through the vertical meridian of the lens exceeds + 1.50 D or so. This formula does not consider factors like the fitting height and the distance power, but still produces satisfactory results in most cases. It is possible to prism thin the minus powered lenses as well. Depending upon the fitting height either base down or base up prism may be required to balance the thickness difference.

We can verify this prism onto the progressive addition lenses by placing the prism reference point of the lens in front of the center of the lens of the focimeter. This is very important especially where only one lens is being replaced. If the previous lens had not been prism thinned and the new one was or vice-versa—an unwanted vertical prism imbalance will be induced. In summary prism thinning is a useful tool that improves both the finished cosmetics of many progressive addition lenses with little visual impact to the wearer.

LIMITATION OF CONVENTIONAL PROGRESSIVE ADDITION LENSES

With all the advancements from hard to soft design and from a required minimum fitting height of 26 mm to 14 mm, many eye care professionals assumed that progressive addition lenses had come relatively close to perfection. However, this is not true. There are still five basic limitations in conventional progressive addition lenses created by their inherent designing.

1. Differing Magnification throughout the Lens

The changing curves on the front lens surface and the change in power throughout the channel and reading portion of the lens create varying magnification throughout the lens **(Fig. 11.31)**. The magnification increases throughout the progressive zone. The result is that the vertical lines viewed through the progression zone exhibit skew distortion **(Fig. 11.32)**.

2. Restricted Visual Field

Progressive addition lens restricts our field of vision particularly for intermediate or near areas. The curves are always on the front side of the conventional progressive addition lenses which position the visual area of the lens at considerably away from the eye. The ultimate result is restriction of visual field.

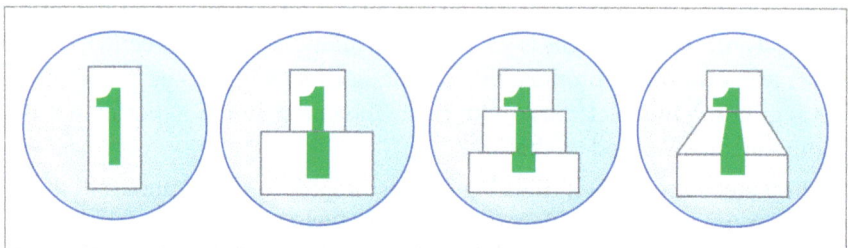

Fig. 11.31: Progressive addition lens magnifies the image in its various section

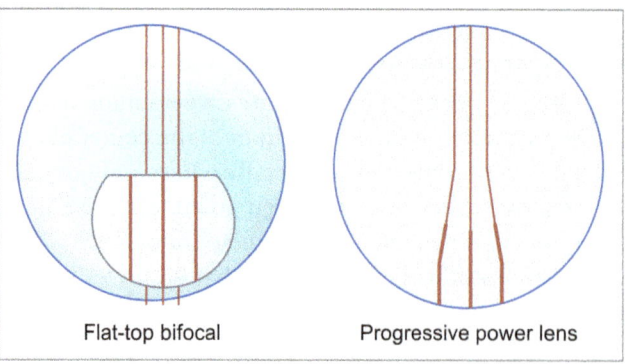

Fig. 11.32: Skewed distortion in a progressive lens

3. Compromised Optics

Conventional progressive addition lenses are produced in varying base curves averaged for a wide range of prescription and a nearest suitable front base curve is used for a given prescription. Ideally the base curve selected should match the exact curves used on the backside. This is simply not possible in conventional progressive addition lenses. As a result acuity is compromised to some extent in all visual areas, depending on how close the front base curve is averaged for the patients prescription.

4. No Control over the Inset of the Near Portion

Some progressive addition lens designs do have an inset, which varies with addition and/or distance correction, but not yet with interpupillary distance.

5. Difficult to check with Focimeters

Progressive addition lenses are relatively difficult to check with the help of focimeter, specially if the original engravings including those indicating distance power circle and near power zone cannot be found.

■ RESTORATION OF PROGRESSIVE ADDITION LENS MARKINGS

Majority of the progressive addition lens manufacturers employ laser etched molds or fluorescent ink markings on the front lens surface to help dispenser identify the lens brands, lens design, addition power, distance power circle and near power circle and thereby enabling the dispenser to fit the lens into the frame properly. These micro engraving, if removed can be detected under a bright light using a dark background. Some manufacturers also provide tools or instruments with appropriate lighting background and magnifier to ease the process of marking restoration.

The first step in identifying a progressive addition lens is to locate the hidden circle or manufacture's symbol located on the 0–180 degree line, 4 mm below the fitting cross on both nasal and temporal sides of the lens. Below these two markings, we find the near addition power (sometimes abbreviated) on the temporal side and the symbol identifying the particular lens on the nasal side. Once the two hidden circles and the brands are identified, place the lens on the respective brand layout card with two circles of the lens coinciding with the two circles on the card and locate the other markings using the layout card as reference.

The following options may be followed:

The micro engraving can be detected by reflecting light from the overhead lights off the lens surface.

Or, fogging the lens surface by breathing warm moist air onto the lens surface.

Or, position the light source behind the lens.

Or, hold the progressive addition lens 10–15 cm in front of the striped grid **(Fig. 11.33)**. Focus on the lens surface.

Or, Using the PAL ID equipment **(Fig. 11.34)**. PAL-ID is a sturdy instrument that illuminate, enlarge and enhance even the faintest engravings on progressive addition lenses. Even the least experienced optician can use it to locate and accurately identify markings in a matter of seconds.

The marking will stand out against the background as shown in the **Figure 11.35**:

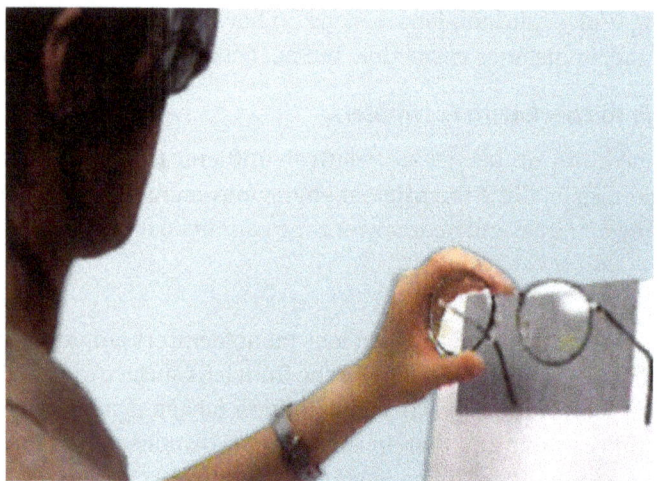

Fig. 11.33: Restoration of progressive lens marking using stripped grid

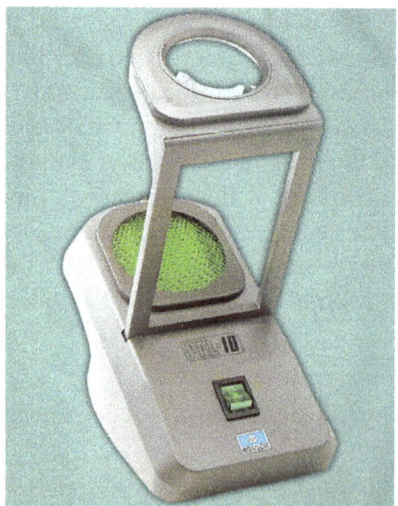

Fig. 11.34: Essilor's PAL ID

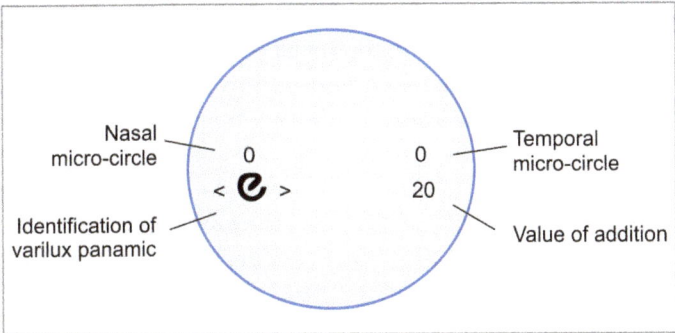

Fig. 11.35: Hidden circles relocated

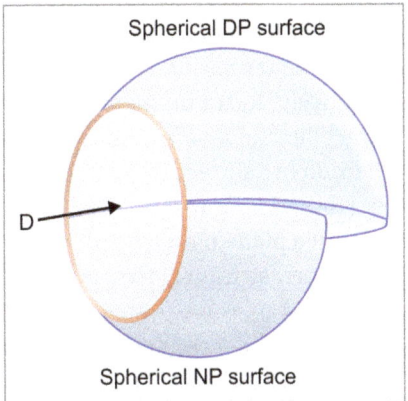

Fig. 11.36: E-style bifocal made by placing together two spherical surfaces with a common tangent at D

GENERATING PROGRESSIVE POWER SURFACE

A progressive power lens surface is an aspheric surface of the non-rotationally symmetric type, generated by means of computer numerically controlled (CNC) machining of either the surface itself or the mould from which the surface may be cast or slumped. The actual geometry of a given progressive lens surface is always regarded as proprietary information of the lens manufacturers. However, some insight into how the design of a surface might proceed can be obtained by the following illustrations:

To understand the geometry of progressive addition lens surface, we need to consider the E-style bifocal with two different spherical surfaces placed together so that their poles share a common tangent at point D, as shown in **Figure 11.36**, where two surfaces are continuous.

At all other points, there is a step between two surfaces, which increases with the increase in distance from the point D. To produce a truly invisible bifocal design, the two surfaces must be blended together such that the DP surface and NP surface are continuous at all point.

A progressive lens may be considered to have a spherical DP and NP surfaces connected by a surface that's tangential and sagittal radii of curvature decrease according to a specific power law between the distance and near zones of the lens. Theoretically, to make a surface with curvature that increases at the correct rate to satisfy the given power law, we need to combine small segments of spheres of ever decreasing radii, all-tangential to one another in a continuous curve. These sections will be continuous only along a single so called meridian or umbilical line and at all other points of the sections; the surface of the sections must be blended to form a smooth surface.

The simplest concept of this can be explained with a section taken from an oblate ellipsoid, as shown in the **Figure 11.37**, where the radii of curvature of the spherical surfaces which represent the distance and near portions are shown as r_D and r_N respectively. It can be seen that the solid ovoid, which is obtained by inserting the ellipsoidal section between the two hemispheres shown in the figure, will result in a surface which has no discontinuities. Along the meridian line, D', a cross section through the surface would be circular and the radii of the circles in a plane parallel with either the distance or near portion circles do indeed decrease from r_D to r_N continuously.

The ability to cut surfaces of such a complex nature was made possible by the use of computer numerically controlled (CNC) grinding machines. The

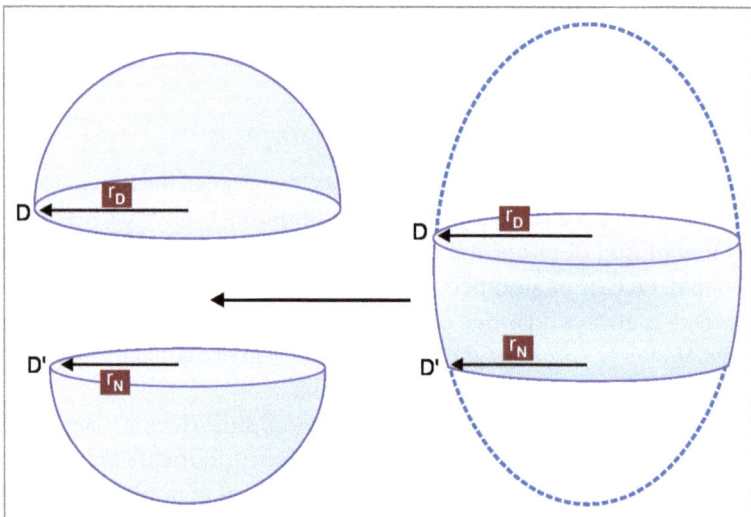

Fig. 11.37: Concept of a progressive lens surface. A section of an oblate ellipsoid is inserted between two hemispheres of radius of curvature r_D for the distance portion and r_N for the near portion

single point diamond tool cuts the surface under computer control, sweeping in an arc over the work piece with the program positioning the cutter in exactly the right place as the cutting tool traverses the work piece.

The work piece could be a glass blank or a glass mould from which plastic lenses might eventually be cast, or it could be a ceramic block upon which glass blanks or finished lens could be slumped with or without vacuum assistance.

The important stages in the production of progressive power surface are as under:
- Surface designing and numeric description.
- Generating the aspheric curve.
- Grinding, smoothing and polishing.
- Inspection.

Surface designing and computation of the surface topography is translated into numeric data in the form of co-ordinates that can be fed directly into the CNC generators. As much as 50000 numeric data point may be required for an individual progressive power surface. The basic reference for the progressive power surface is usually taken to be the spherical surface of curvature required for DP curve. Then the spherical curve is subsequently made aspheric in accordance with the design philosophy for the lens. Before that the spherical convex surface must be smoothed and polished accurately so that its topography has precisely the known desired characteristics.

CNC diamond tool is used to create the aspheric surface as explained earlier. If the work piece is glass blank, it must be smoothed and polished, using floating pad system. It is essential to ensure that the pads do not remove any more glass material than intended; otherwise an accurate surface geometry will not be maintained.

Ceramic slumping moulds produced by CNC cutters can be used to produce progressive power surface. The glass blanks are placed on ceramic moulds as shown in the **Figure 11.38**. The entire assembly is then heated to the high temperature at which the glass starts to flow.

The glass slumps and the geometry of the convex surface of the mould is transferred to convex surface of the blank. The entire process has to be done under highly sophisticated temperature control to ensure that the glass flows correctly. Slumping can be assisted by vacuum forming also, whereby the glass is heated to just beyond its softening point, whereupon, a vacuum is applied to the interface between the forming block and the concave surface of the blank—which pulls the surface into shape.

It is the dream of the lens designer to create a progressive addition lens with no areas of distortions at the either side of the lens, which unfortunately is just not possible. The distortion on the either side is the result of induced cylinder, which is due to the presence of unwanted surface astigmatism and is evident

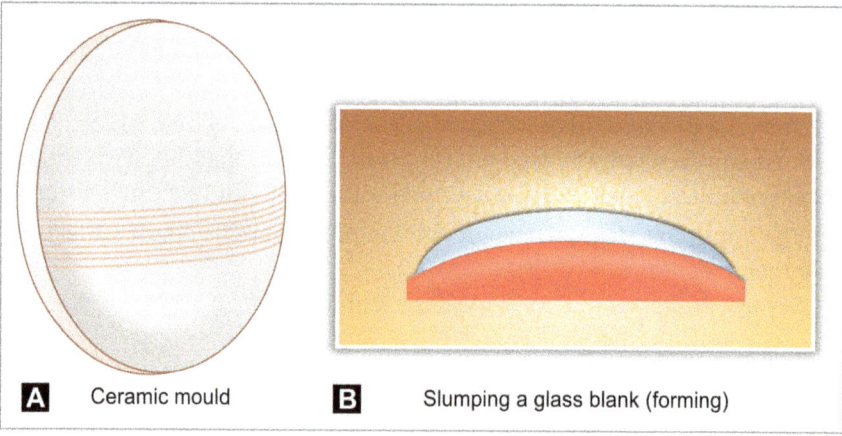

| A | Ceramic mould | B | Slumping a glass blank (forming) |

Fig. 11.38: Slumping a glass blank to a required geometry

during the lateral gaze within the progressive zone. All that the designer can do is to reduce distortions to the minimum. Progressive designs vary from one to another only by how these "no go" areas of the lens are distributed across its surface.

The astigmatism across the pupil is inversely proportional to the length of the progression zone. The longer is the progression zone, the smaller is the surface astigmatism. In other words the rate of change in the surface astigmatism in the periphery depends upon the addition. Higher addition gives faster changes and hence peripheral astigmatism is more evident.

The reduction of peripheral distortion is also accomplished by using the conic sections of changing asphericity rather than spherical sections as power is increased in the vertical meridian. These varying sections reach a relatively uniform power at a given peripheral portion of the lenses so that prismatic and cylindrical effect at these edges are much the same through out the peripheral vertical range of the lens. To achieve this in the upper portion, the distance section is increased slightly in power towards the periphery by + 0.30 D. This type of design also reduces the "optically pure" zone for near in width by allowing the reduced remaining power variation to spread over more area. As the curves are aspherical, the near zone reveals a spherical area of only 12 mm wide. However, the power change is so gradual that a much wider defective zone of practically equivalent power exists, depending upon the power of addition.

EVOLUTION OF PROGRESSIVE ADDITION LENS

The first commercially successful progressive addition lens was introduced by Essel under the name of Varilux in 1959. The design consisted of large spherical distance and near zones, linked by a series of circles of ever decreasing radii between the distance vision sphere and the near vision sphere. More attention had been given to ensure larger distance and near zones than to the quality of peripheral vision on either side of the progressive corridor as shown in **Figure 11.39**. Today such a design would be described as very hard design.

The second generation of progressive lenses, Varilux 2 was introduced in 1973. It too provided large distance, intermediate and near fields of vision, but still it was at the cost of quality vision in the lateral regions of the progressive zone. Conic sections of changing eccentricities from one section of the lens to another replaced the circular section employed in Varilux 1 design. The effect of this was the reduction of power in the periphery of the progressive zone. The new concept of "horizontal optical modulation" was introduced which took care of the extra-foveal vision also. Binocular vision was optimized as a result of an asymmetrical design. The overall design of the lens is represented by a succession of conic sections as shown in the **Figure 11.40**.

During the next decade other manufacturer introduced progressive addition lens design focusing specific optical characteristics. Some emphasized on large distance and near vision zones, concentrating the inevitable astigmatism in the lens periphery. American Optical Ultravue, Rodenstock Progressive R, Sola Graduate etc., were in this category. Other manufacturer took a different approach, reducing the amount of unwanted astigmatism in the periphery by spreading it more widely in the lens. Truvision Omni of American Optical became popular. Zeiss Gradal HS placed special emphasis on the concept of the lens asymmetry and comfortable binocular vision.

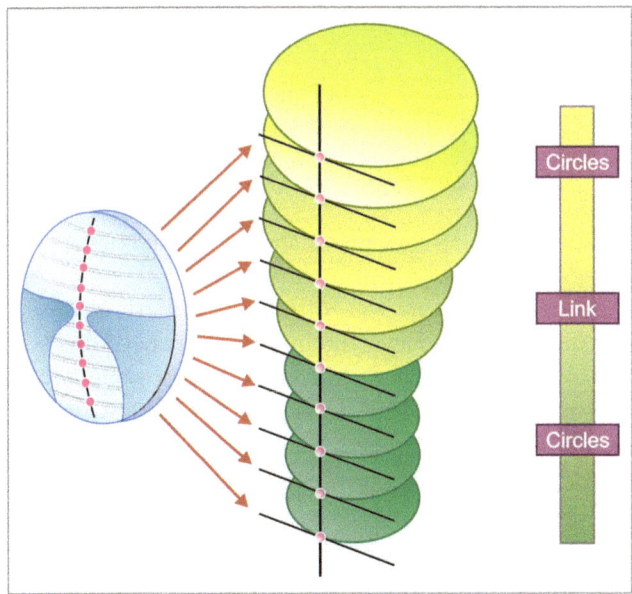

Fig. 11.39: First progressive addition lens

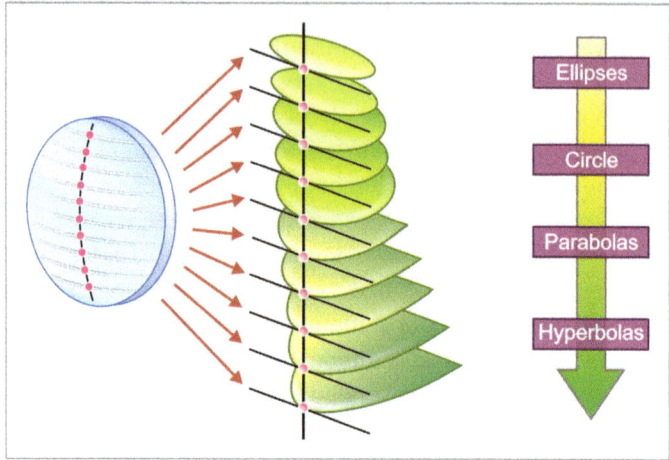

Fig. 11.40: The "Physiological" progressive addition lens

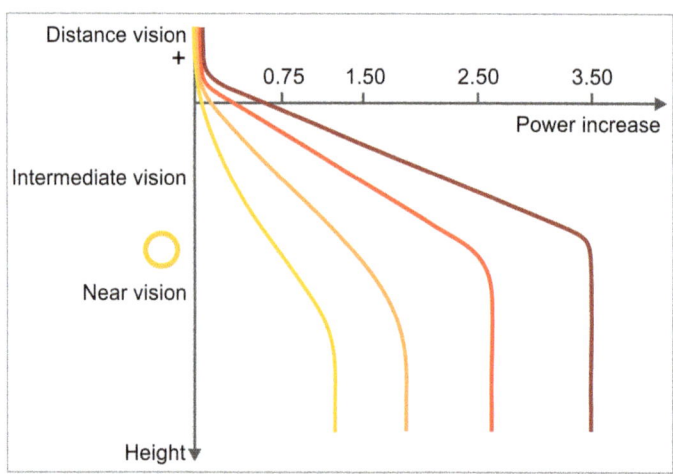

Fig. 11.41: Multi-design progressive addition lens

Soon multi-design concept was introduced in Varilux Infinity in 1988 – the third generation progressive. The multi-design used district designs to match the wearers changing needs with advancing presbyopia. Multi-design concept refers to the change of power progression profile with near addition, generally resulting in a larger progression length for a low addition and hence soft design. The corridor length becomes shorter and the design harder as the addition increases. The multi design concept is well illustrated with the change of power progression profile by addition in the **Figure 11.41**.

Essilor introduced the fourth generation of progressive lenses under the brand name of Varilux Comfort in 1993, which offered more natural vision than any previous progressive lens designs. The near vision area in this lens design is located high, so that the wearer can reach it easily and naturally when lowering their gaze. Fewer head and eye movement are required to explore the near and intermediate vision fields and hence the wearer enjoys more comfortable posture. These advantages were because of specific power profile in the progression zone adopted for Varilux Comfort. For example in case of + 2.00 D addition, 85% of the full addition is reached just 12 mm below the fitting cross compared to a minimum of 14 mm or 15 mm for previous progressive designs. Due to the softness in the lens periphery, the wearer enjoys additional comfort in the peripheral and dynamic vision as the necessary horizontal head movement required to explore the full of the field was greatly reduced. The asymmetry design incorporated also offered balanced binocular vision, while at the same time integrating the multi design concept of previous progressive lens design. Several competitive designs from other manufacturer appeared during the decade.

In 2002, the fifth generation progressive design – "Varilux Panamic" was introduced. This new design was based on the success achieved by Varilux Comfort in providing a larger field of vision, which resulted from the softness and regularity of the lens periphery. The Varilux Comfort design showed that the vision was a global process and the wearer would perceive their field as larger if they had the ability to see comfortably through the lens periphery. In the Varilux Panamic design, the balance between the control zone and the periphery was shifted towards the peripheral zone of the lens, so that peripheral effect were lens dramatic than the previous designs. This change also brought the advantages of reducing the swimming effects obtained by rotation of the head and eyes around the field and improving binocular fusion in the lens periphery. Clinical trials have found significant enlargement in the field of vision in all zones of the lens.

New generation designs from other manufacturers include the BBGR Evolis, the Nikon Presio W, the Pentex Super Atoric F, the Seiko P-ISY—the first of the new designs to have the progression on the concave surface, Hoya's Hoyalux D design, is double sided progressive.

The most recent development in the progressive addition lenses is the Varilux Ipseo from Essilor—the personalized progressive lens that takes into account the actual degree of head and eye movement which the wearer employs when viewing through the intermediate and near zones of the lens. Research has been shown that each individual has specific head and eye behavior, which can be measured and then the progressive surface is designed to incorporate the wearers behavior.

Over the last few years rapid strides have taken place in ophthalmic lens production technology. Through a combination of better software, faster computer processing and free form surfacing, it has become possible to modify some aspects a progressive design to take into account the individual characteristic of the frame in which the lenses are to be mounted.

CURRENT PROGRESSIVE LENS DESIGN DEVELOPMENT

With the changing scenario in the trend of spectacle dispensing, lot of new development have come in progressive addition lens designing, with special regard to the followings:

Shorter Corridor Progressive Lens (Fig. 11.42)

When the progressive lenses were, first introduced, the recommended minimum fitting height was 22 mm. That was fine when the eye sizes of the spectacle frames were large and had deep 'B' measurements. However, as the smaller and narrower frame shapes become popular, a need for progressive with shorter corridor was crucial to their continued success. Smaller frames proportions differ from large frames in that they have a higher horizontal to vertical ratio. In other words the lens has to be not only shorter vertically but also relatively wider. The second challenge is to provide distortion free distance vision in the lens periphery. Finally the shorter corridor lens must account for the fact that the wearer's head and eye movement are influenced by frame size. Wearer of small frames tend to move their head more and eyes less when transitioning from distance to near viewing than that of large frame wearers. When looking down a short corridor lens, the eyes simply run out of the lens, so the head has to move to maintain focus on the items of regard.

To make the progressive addition lens work in small frames, many lens manufacturers came out with shorter corridor progressives. In 1999, American Optical introduced AO Compact—the first short corridor progressive lens. AO Compact has a 13 mm corridor that permits full reading function with a minimum fitting height of 17 mm. Soon other companies followed the suit and shorter corridor progressive becomes popular: Nikon Presio, Essilor Ellipse, Shamir Piccolo, Hoya Hoyalux Summit CD, Kodak Concise, Pentex Mini AF, etc., became popular.

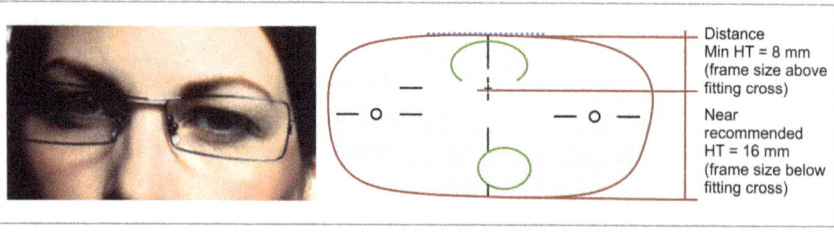

Fig. 11.42: A typical shorter corridor progressive

Internal Progressive

Internal progressive addition lens is a big step forward in overcoming many of the limitations of progressive lenses widely available today. Seiko is proud to have designed and patented the world's first internal progressive lenses. In an internal progressive lens, the curves producing changing power are positioned on the back surface of the lens, and front surface is spherical. The backside is a free form surface with progressive surface and cylinder surface on the back. Therefore, it is possible to have a spherical front curve. The design provides a field of vision that is 30% wider than a front side progressive lens. This is due to the fact that the progressive surface rests closer to the eyes. Besides Seiko, Rodenstock ILT is also being test marketed in the USA. The new internal design offers following additional advantages:
- Expansion of the visual fields
- Magnification differences between various areas of the lens are reduced.

Customized Progressives

Customized or personalized or individualized progressive surface design is the most unique and the latest development in the progressive addition lenses. The latest design from Essilor's Ipseo takes into account the actual degree of head and eye rotation that the wearer employs when viewing through the intermediate and near zones of the lens. Research has shown that each individual has specific head and eye movement behavior, which can be measured and the progressive surface can be designed to incorporate the wearer's behavior. This principle has been incorporated into the personalized progressive design from Essilor-the Varilux Ipseo.

A new instrument the vision print system as shown in the **Figure 11.43**, has been developed to determine eye/head movement for a specific individual, the

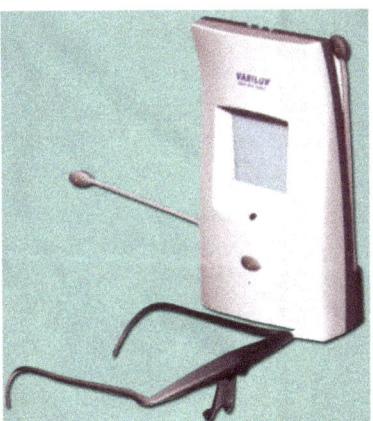

Fig. 11.43: Vision print system

result of which can be incorporated into the progressive surface. The system consists of three lamps – the central lamp is viewed at 40 cms from the center of the wearers forehead, with two separate lamps, 40 cms on either side of the central lamp. The wearer is directed to look at the lamp, which is illuminated and their head movement is recorded by an ultrasonic signal that is emitted by the system and reflected by a transponder attached to the special trial frame the wearer is wearing. As far as the wearer is concerned, the lamps are illuminated at random following a short 15 second cycle and it continuous over a 90 second cycle which enables the systems to calculate and display the eye/head movement ratio, along with a consistency factor referred to as the "Stability co-efficient" (ST). ST is used to adjust the rate of transition between the central and peripheral zones of the lens. Most people's eye/head ratio is relatively stable, having stability co-efficient below 0.15. ST value 0.00 shows the high stability of head and eyes movement. The indicator A in the instrument indicates head/eye proportion, the number at B shows the head/eye movement ratio and the number at point C shows the stability co-efficient. The number 0.31 in the **Figure 11.44** reflects that the subject is performing 31% of the gaze movement with their head and 69% with their eyes. The ST of 0.07 indicates high stability of the head and eye movement behavior.

The eye mover uses more of the surface of the lens, so they need a larger acuity zone. For them the harder design as shown in the **Figure 11.45** can be

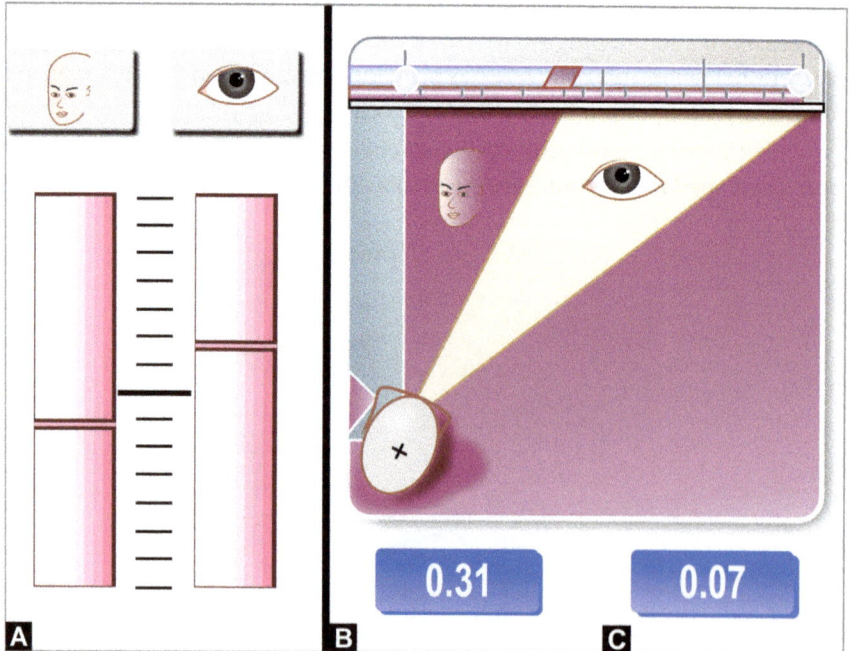

Fig. 11.44: The information displayed on the screen

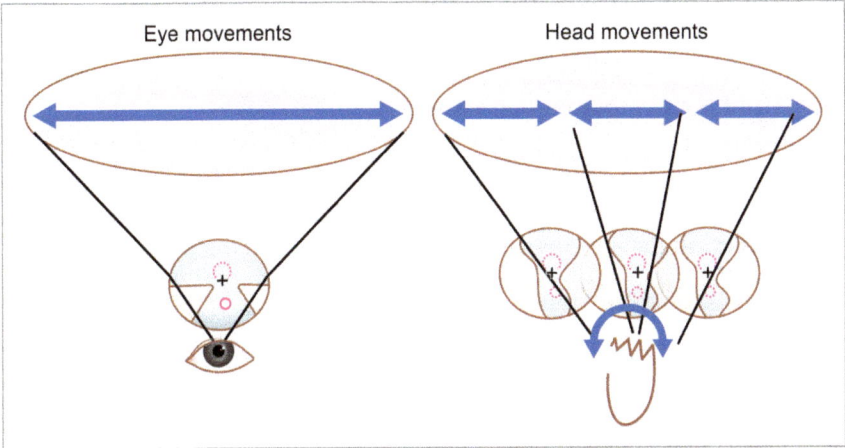

Fig. 11.45: Studies show that the head-eye movement ratio directly influences the area of the lens that is used by the wearer

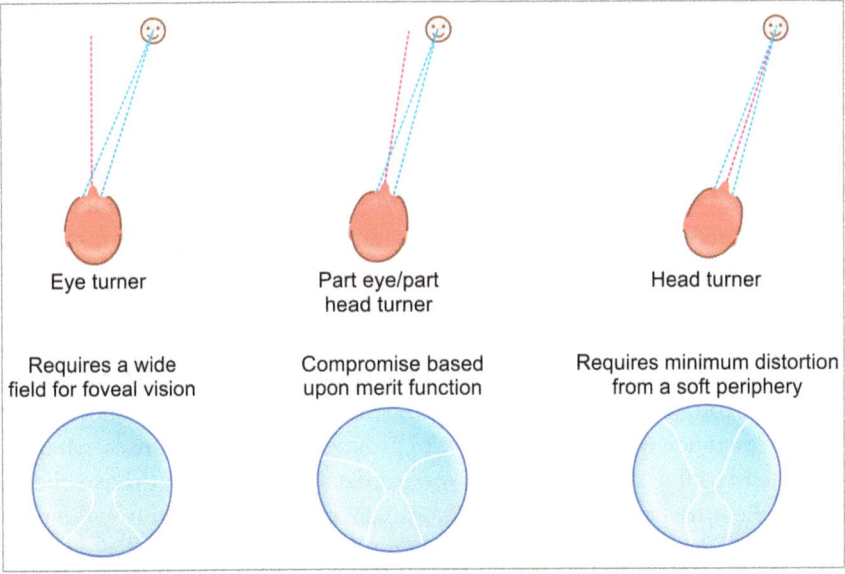

Fig. 11.46: Progressive designs for eye turners and head turners

more useful. On the other hand the "head-mover", having more dynamic vision, will be more influenced by the periphery of the lens as their head moves in their visual world and will be benefited from the peripheral "softness" as shown in the **Figure 11.46**. Each Varilux Ipseo lens is designed for the individual wearer, manufactured by free-form technology and to recognize its individual nature, micro-engraved with the wearers initials.

WHO IS SUITABLE FOR PROGRESSIVE ADDITION LENSES?
(Criteria for good candidate)

The introduction of numerous varieties of progressive lenses has made it suitable for almost every presbyopes, for every visual demand and for every wallets, Still proper selection of an ideal candidate is the first criteria for the successful dispensing of progressive addition lens. Before identifying a suitable candidate, the evaluation must be done on the following factors:

General Considerations

Careful consideration is needed before advising progressive addition lenses for those with any history of difficulties in adapting to changes in lens power or frame styles. Persons having an interest in trying new things can be good candidates. People with small pupil are more suitable for progressive addition lenses as the effect of peripheral aberration is reduced. An unsatisfied patient with other designs of bifocals may found himself motivated to adjust with progressive lenses. The patient with narrow pupillary distance and wider facial width may also be an unsatisfied user of progressive lenses.

Visual Needs

Information about the patients visual needs enables the practitioner to understand whether the progressive addition lenses will meet the patient expectations or not. Those who require a larger field of view can immediately be eliminated from the consideration. An avid user of computers will be benefited more by occupational lenses rather than a progressive addition lenses. The progressive addition lenses for him may be prescribed as a supplement for general use. Most commonly used near working distance also influence the selection criteria. A patient who invariably works at shorter and middle distance will be a happy user of progressive addition lenses, whereas a constant user of shorter reading, working distance will prefer to have bifocal lenses. Relative use for distance/near visual zones also sometimes influences the criteria. Myopes who depend more on distance visual zone have always been more successful user of progressive lenses.

Refractive Status

Progressive addition lenses should be avoided for that refraction which may induce vertical prism between the eyes including different refraction between the eyes by more than 2.00 D in spherical power or more than 2.00 D in effective cylinder power especially in the vertical meridian (horizontal axis).

IDEAL FRAME SELECTION FOR PROGRESSIVE ADDITION LENS

The ideal frame selection is an important criterion for the successful dispensing of progressive addition lenses. Many a times it has been seen that in spite of having perfect refraction and fitting, the patient is not the happy user of the progressive lenses and the reason established is not other than poor frame selection. The frame should be selected in such a manner so as to cover adequate facial width and also minimizes the vertex distance. Metal frames with adjustment nose pad are more suitable than plastic frames as the fitting height can be adjusted, if required, using the nose pads. While selecting the suitable frame for an individual who is opting for progressive addition lens, the following two factors must be taken into consideration.

Shape of the Frames

Square and panto shapes as shown in the **Figures 11.47 and 11.48** are the most suitable shapes for the progressive addition lenses. Steep rectangular shapes extending beyond the temporal bone of the face may not be suitable. Another important factor in frame selection is ensuring that the shape of the frame does not reduce the size of the reading area by being too "cut away" in the nasal area of the frame. For example, an aviator shape frame **(Fig. 11.49)** coupled with narrow pupillary distance may present such a difficulty.

Size/Depth of the Frame

The frame must have sufficient depth **(Fig. 11.50)** to accommodate the entire zones of the progressive lens from the top of the distance power circle to the bottom of the near power circle within its aperture, i.e., the 'B' measurement should be adequate to include full distance and near optical zones. Another important factor, which is usually overlooked, is the 'A'-measurement of the frame, i.e., it must minimize the distance between the position of the fitting cross and the temporal end of the frame.

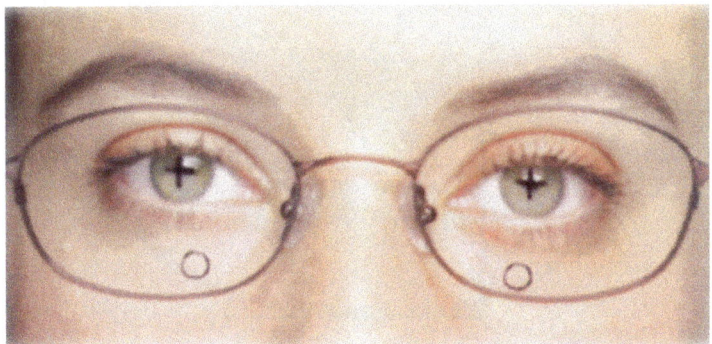

Fig. 11.47: Ideal square shape of frame for progressive addition lens

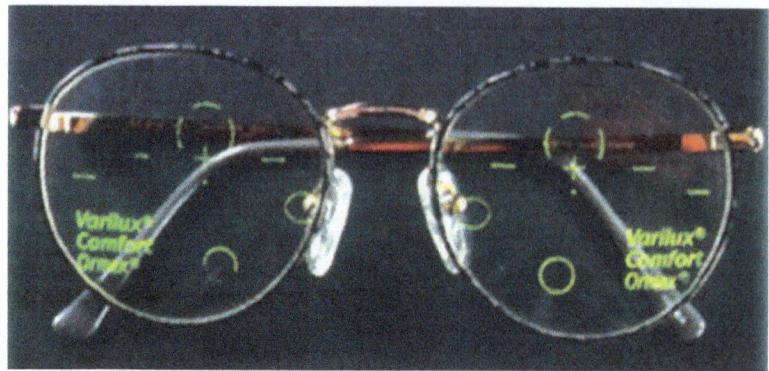

Fig. 11.48: Ideal panto shape of frame for progressive addition lens

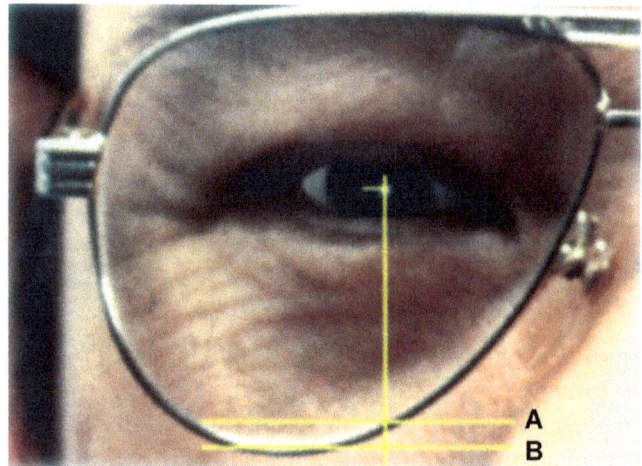

Fig. 11.49: Aviator shape cuts away the reading area in the nasal side

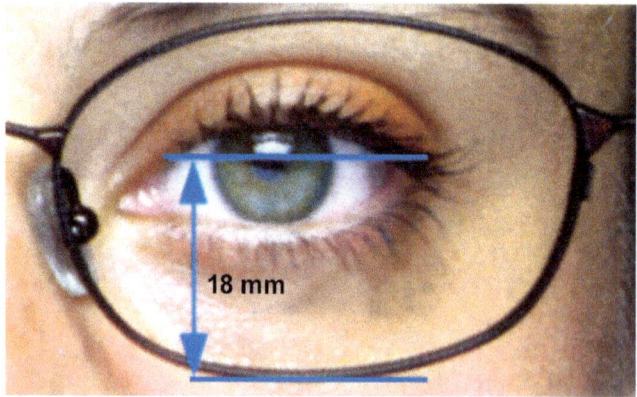

Fig. 11.50: Sufficient height between the pupil and the lower rim of the frame

Once the lenses are properly marked and verified on the wearer's face, the layout card can be used to ensure the confirmation of above factors.

DISPENSING PROGRESSIVE ADDITION LENSES

Progressive lenses should be centered with respect to the eye so that the vision zone can be used ideally at all distance. The fitting of progressive lenses should be carried out with normal, relaxed head and body position and with the eyes looking horizontally straight ahead. The fitting can be done using manual measurement. But before that it is important that you fit the selected frame on the wearers face and then take the measurement. The following adjustment needs to be confirmed:

Frame Front Adjustment (Fig. 11.51)

Adjust the angle of the temples so that the frame sits squarely on the face.

Pantoscopic Tilt (Fig. 11.52)

Adjust temples to achieve 8 to 12 degrees tilt, avoid contact with cheeks.

Facial Wrap (Fig. 11.53)

Ensure that the front of the frame follows the line of the face but not excessively.

Temple Length (Fig. 11.54)

Adjust length of temple to minimize sliding.

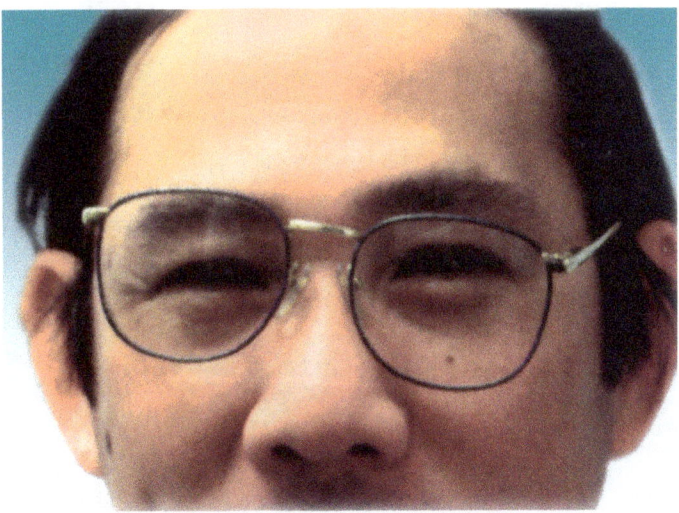

Fig. 11.51: Front of the frame not in alignment

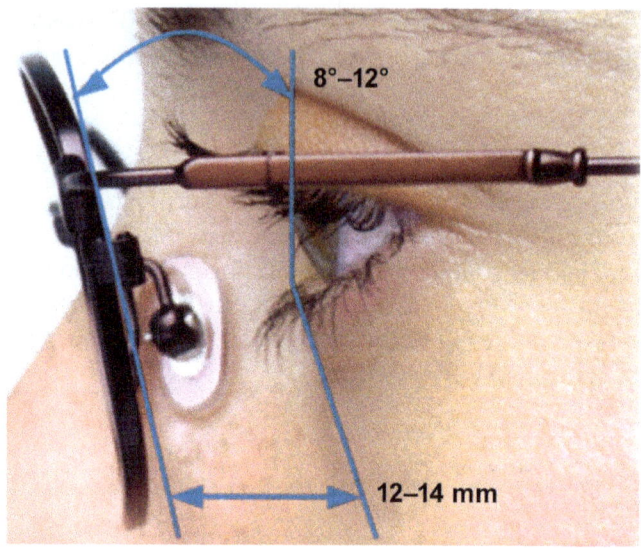

Fig. 11.52: 8 to 10 degree pantoscopic tilt

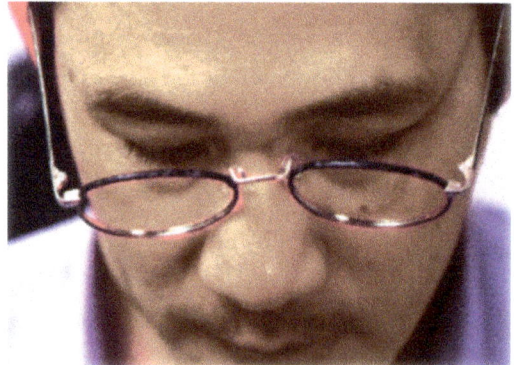

Fig. 11.53: Poor facial wrap

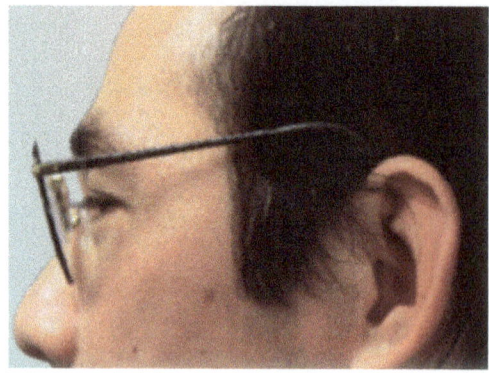

Fig. 11.54: Needs to lengthen side bend

Vertex Distance

Minimize Vertex distance by adjusting nose pads but avoid contacting the eyelashes with the lens.

Once the above adjustment are done, take the following two measurement:
1. Monocular PD for distance
2. Fitting height

Monocular PD for Distance

The monocular PD is the distance from the center of the nose bridge to the center of the pupil, specified to the nearest 0.5 mm. A number of devices can be used to measure monocular PD:
- Pupillometer **(Fig. 11.55)**
- PD Ruler **(Fig. 11.56)**
- Marking directly on the lens insert

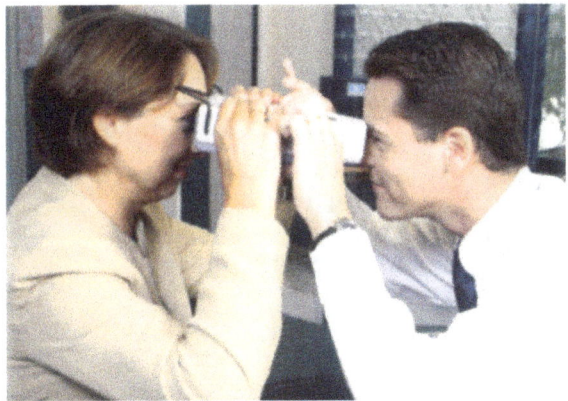

Fig. 11.55: Measuring PD with pupillometer

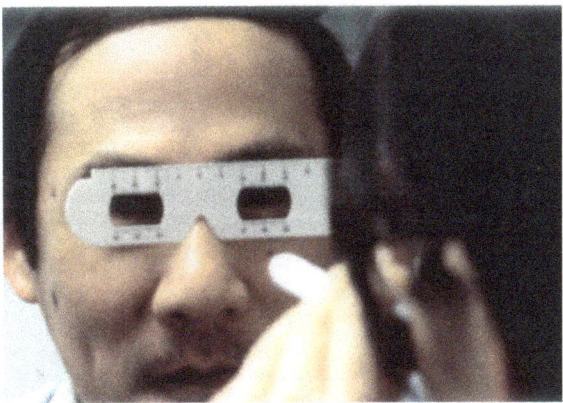

Fig. 11.56: Measuring monocular PD with ruler

After determining the monocular PD, mark their location on the lens insert in the following ways:
- Place the frame symmetrically and level on the progressive addition lens layout card.
- At the determined PD, mark a vertical line on each lens insert **(Fig. 11.57)**.
- Place the frame back on the wearers face to check the accuracy of PD **(Fig. 11.58)**.

Fitting Height

The fitting cross on progressive addition lens must coincide with the pupil center of the wearers in their natural posture. The position of the pupil center relative to the correctly adjusted frame is the fitting height, and is specified as the distance above the deepest point of the inner frame rim to the nearest 1 mm. Occasionally some practitioners prefer to specify the fitting height as mm above datum, which is the line halfway between the uppermost and lowermost rims of the frame.

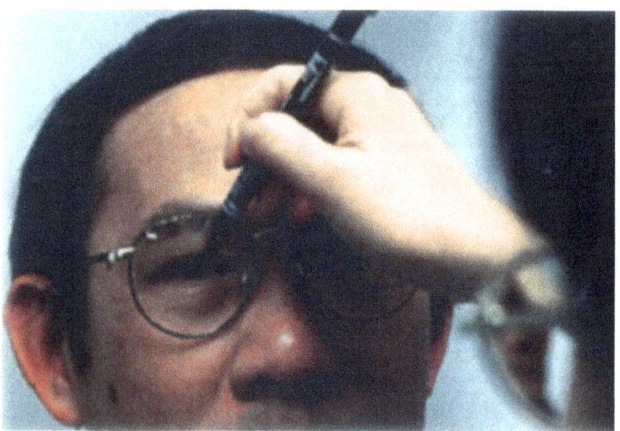

Fig. 11.57: Marking on the lens inserts

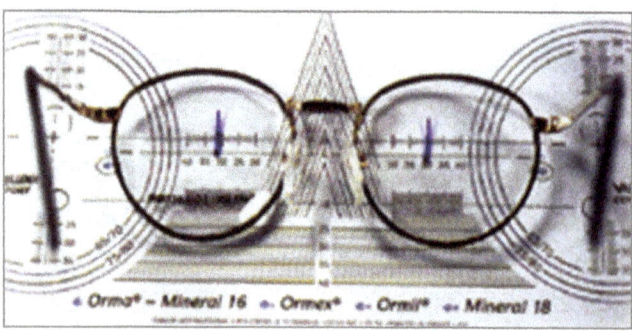

Fig. 11.58: Marking vertical lines on the layout

The following procedure is used to measure the fitting height **(Fig. 11.59)**:
- Place yourself opposite and at the same height as the wearer.
- Ask the wearer to adopt a comfortable posture and look straight ahead.
- Ask the wearer to look at your LE.
- Hold a pen torch just below your LE.
- Close your RE to avoid parallax error.
- Observe the position of the light reflection in the wearers RE relative to the vertical PD line already marked on the lens.
- Place a small horizontal mark on the PD line corresponding to the pupil center **(Fig. 11.60)**.

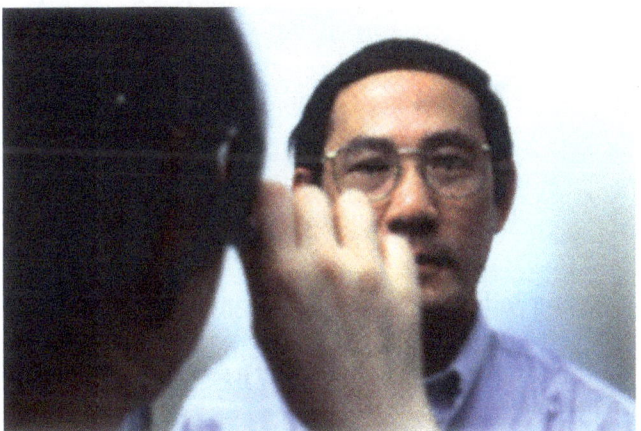

Fig. 11.59: Fitting height measurement

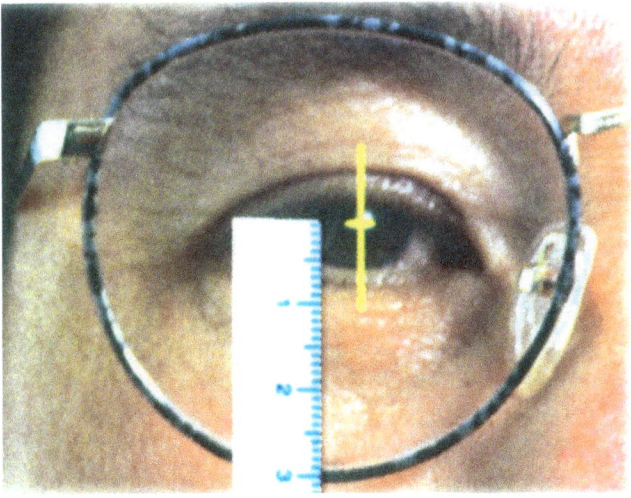

Fig. 11.60: Fitting height measurement (29 mm in this picture)

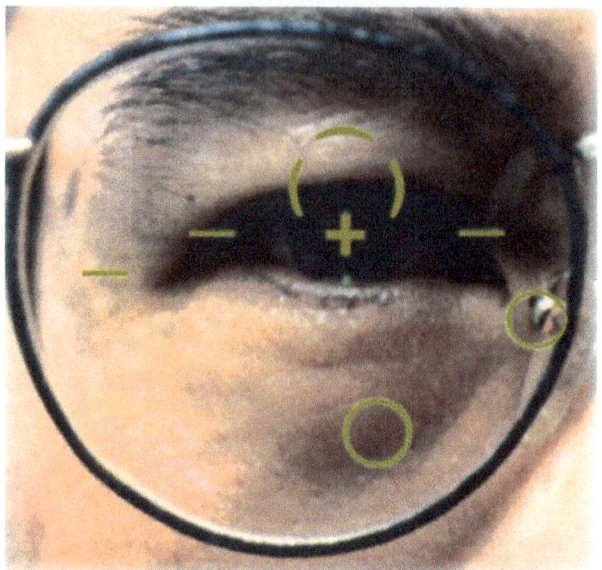

Fig. 11.61: Ideal position of the fitting cross

- Ask the wearer to look at your RE and complete the procedure for the other eye.
- Move the frame up and down slightly, let it settle, and report for both eyes.
- Confirm the final marked lens insert.

The ideal position of the fitting cross should be as shown in the **Figure 11.61**.

Multiple Choice Questions (MCQs)

1. Which of the following is true of fitting cross point when we talk about progressive addition lens?
    a. It is the top end of the corridor length
    b. Astigmatism starts perpendicular to this point on either side
    c. The fitting cross represents the alignment point of the lens design
    d. All of the above

2. At which of the following position the base curve of the progressive addition lens can be checked using Geneva Lens measure?
    a. Distance reference point
    b. Prism reference point
    c. Near reference point
    d. All of the above

Chapter 11: Progressive Addition Lenses

3. Prism thinning involves adding…..
   a. Base up prism
   b. Base down prism
   c. Base out prism
   d. Base in prism

4. Where should prism be measured on a progressive power lens?
   a. Midway between the horizontal alignment engravings
   b. 1.5 mm below the fitting cross
   c. At the fitting cross
   d. Where the add is engraved

5. For which types of progressive lens prescriptions will the maximum benefits of prism-thinning be seen?
   a. High positive distance powers with high additions
   b. Low negative distance powers with high additions
   c. High positive distance powers with low additions
   d. Plano prescriptions with high additions

6. As the add power of a progressive lens increases, the unwanted cylinder power typically:
   a. Decreases
   b. Increases
   c. Remains unchanged
   d. Disappears

7. The amount of prism thinning applied to a lens is dependent on………..
   a. The frame style
   b. The add power
   c. The lens refractive index
   d. The position of the fitting cross

8. Mono design progressive addition lens is characterized by:
   a. Position for near vision does not change with the change in near addition
   b. Both right and left lens have similar design
   c. One single curve along the vertical length of the corridor
   d. All of the above

9. Multi design progressive addition lens is characterized by:
   a. Position for near vision changes with the change in near addition
   b. Both right and left lens have asymmetry design
   c. Multiple curve along the distance viewing zone
   d. All of the above

Answers

1. d   2. a   3. b   4. a   5. a   6. b   7. b   8. a   9. a

Chapter 12

Safety Lenses

Studies show that there is unacceptably large number of eye injuries occurring in the world. The visual impairment as a result of an eye injury may vary from a slight reduction in visual acuity to the total blindness. In the past these eye injuries have been associated with industrial occupations only but now there are increasing number of eye injuries seen in sports, leisure activities and at home also. All such ocular hazards caused by eye injuries can be divided into two groups as shown in **Figure 12.1**:
1. Mechanical
2. Non-mechanical.

Mechanical injuries may arise from a variety of causes and their effects are generally divided into two main categories—contusion and perforation. Contusion injury may result from various causes including flying blunt objects, falling objects, explosions or compressed air accidents, fluids under pressure escaping from burst pipes and water jets from fire hoses. The effects of contusion on the various ocular structures are numerous. It may lead to black eye, subconjunctival hemorrhage, corneal abrasion, blow out fracture, hyphema, iridodialysis, cataract, choroidal ruptures, scleral ruptures, angle recession, retinal hemorrhage etc., perforating ocular injuries can be caused by foreign bodies.

Non-mechanical ocular injuries fall into four main categories—chemical, thermal, electrical and radiation. Most chemicals harm the eyes by direct contact with the external ocular tissues. Concentrated sulphuric acid from exploding car batteries, household bleaches, detergents, disinfectants and lime are examples of chemicals that can cause burns to the eyes. Thermal injuries can be caused by flames and contact burns. Hot bodies, fluids or gases are the usual sources. Burns usually involve the eyelids and not the globe, which is

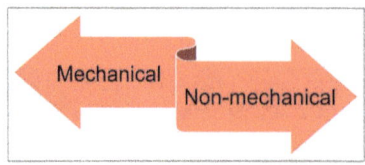

Fig. 12.1: Ocular hazards

often protected by reflex blink. Electrical injuries are basically due to lighting and high tension electrical appliances. Injuries to eyebrows, eyelashes with superficial burns of lids which are usually associated with marked swelling and conjunctival chemosis are hazards caused by electrical injuries. Radiation injuries involve damage to the eyes as a result of absorption of harmful radiation. UV radiation can affect both the skin and the eyes. Pingeculae, pterygium and band shaped keratopathies are thought to be caused partially by long term chronic exposure to UV radiation. Cataracts are also thought to be caused by absorption of UV radiation. Visible light may also cause damage by thermal photocoagulation. Retinal burns may occur when high intensities of light are focused on the retina. Infrared radiation, when absorbed, leads to thermal effect on the tissue.

These ocular hazards are associated not only with industrial occupations, but also with sports, leisure activities are on the increase. In USA, the greatest number of injuries results from base ball, ice hockey and racket sports. Racket sports are responsible for many ocular injuries, and this is not surprising, given the speed of the ball. A squash ball may reach speed of 224 km/hour, a tennis ball 192 km/hour and a shuttlecock 232 km/hour. There is also the risk of the player being hit by the opponent's racket. Many severe ocular injuries occur to children at play and in the home and at times such accidents become the major cause of blindness.

Many of such ocular hazards can be prevented by widespread use of eye protectors in the form of safety glasses. Tinted lenses protect the eyes from harmful radiations. It may also be necessary to protect the eyes against the other ocular hazards, arising from dust, flying particles, industrial environment, sports injuries etc. Legislation is now there to protect the eyes both in the work environment and in certain sports, such as squash and protection may need to be provided, whether the lenses include a refractive correction or not, in the form of safety glasses.

Safety glasses provide protection against impact, chemical or molten metal splashes, dust or radiations from welding arcs of lasers. It may take the form of spectacles, goggles, visors, face shields or hoods. Good safety glasses are made from polycarbonate and are shatter resistant. This does not mean they are unbreakable or that they will last for ever. Their purpose is to protect the wearer from injury from accidental projectiles and particles. As the lenses become exposed to more and more bits and pieces of materials over time, they will become pitted. The more pitted they become, the less clear the wearer will be able to see things. More importantly, after a while, the bombardment of particles will weaken the lens and they should be replaced. Most safety glasses also provide a high level of UV protection and therefore, can be used as sunglasses.

When you look for safety glasses, there are a number of things to be considered:
- Ensure that the safety eyewear meets the standards applicable for your region and also usage. In USA "ANSI Z 87" should be marked on the frame and the manufacturer's initials and any special lens attribute should be noted on the lens.
- Look for the safety glasses made with high quality, virgin resin polycarbonate material. Recycled resins are cheaper, but they are also burdened with a high degree of distortion and yellowing lenses are not as durable.
- Zero distortion lenses allow you to not only see more clearly through the safety glasses, but also allow you to wear them for longer periods of time without eyestrain or fatigue.
- If you wear the safety glasses over top of your prescription lenses or reading glasses, make sure that they are large enough to fit. Safety glasses with bifocal lenses are available, sometimes allowing you to take off your prescription glasses altogether.
- Fit is very important. There are a few aspects to this—width of the frame, width of the nosepiece, length of the temples and angle of the temple with respect to the lenses.
- Fit ensures comfort, but additional features can enhance this. If the nosepiece is soft, rather than a molded in part of the lens, it will enhance comfort. If the glasses have soft pieces on the temple tips, they will be easier on your ears. If the temple frame is thinner and more flexible, that also adds to comfort. Lastly, if the glasses are lighter in weight, that will help ensure a comfortable wear.
- Replacement lenses, if they are available, can help reduce ongoing costs. However, for most styles of safety glasses, the most expensive component is the lens, so don't expect to be paying a lot less for just the lens.
- Degree of protection is more important than just the safety rating. So the glasses can have the added features of side shields, wrap-around lenses and brow guards.
- Lastly make sure the lens tint is applicable for your specific application.

LENS MATERIALS

The lenses for safety eyewear may be made of different materials as shown in **Flowchart 12.1**.

Flowchart 12.1: Different types of materials used for safety eye wears

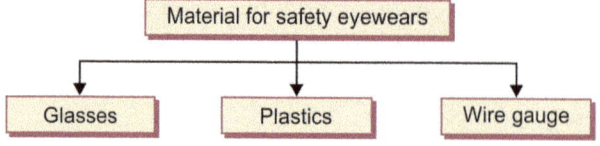

Glasses

Safety glasses may be of different types as shown in **Flowchart 12.2**.

Laminated Glasses

Laminated glass lenses are made by the adhesion of two layers of crown glasses to an inner layer of plastic material as shown in **Figure 12.2**. These lenses are not very strong, but are able to withstand significantly more impact than a standard glass lens. When broken, however, they tend to remain intact as the particles generally adhered to the center plastic layer as shown in **Figure 12.3**.

Heat Toughened Glasses

Heat toughened glass lenses are usually made from spectacle crown glass. The toughening process begins when the edged lens is placed in a furnace and heated to 637°C for 50–300 seconds. The time spent in the oven depends on the weight, size and average thickness of the lens. After heating, the lens is

Flowchart 12.2: Different types of safety glasses

- Laminated glasses
- Heat toughened glasses
- Chemically toughened glasses
- Special heat toughened safety glasses

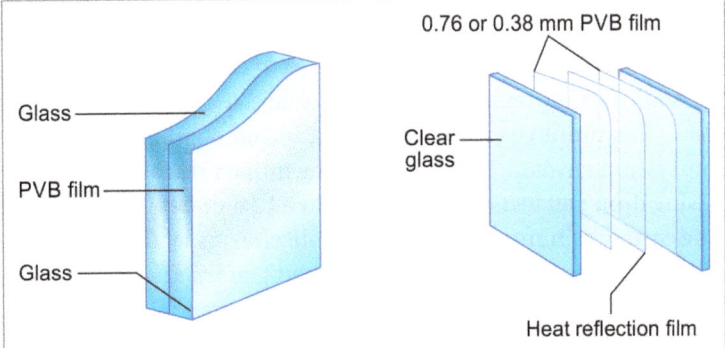

Fig. 12.2: PVC film is sandwiched between two glass surfaces of a laminated glass

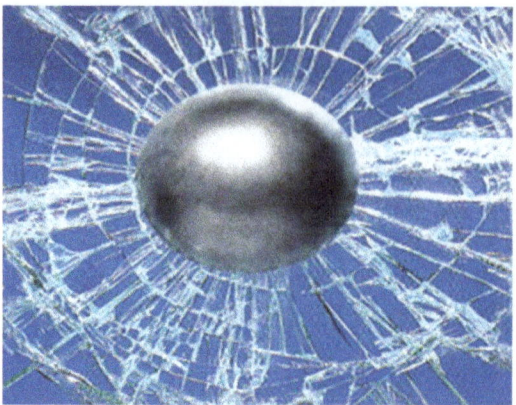

Fig. 12.3: Broken laminated glass

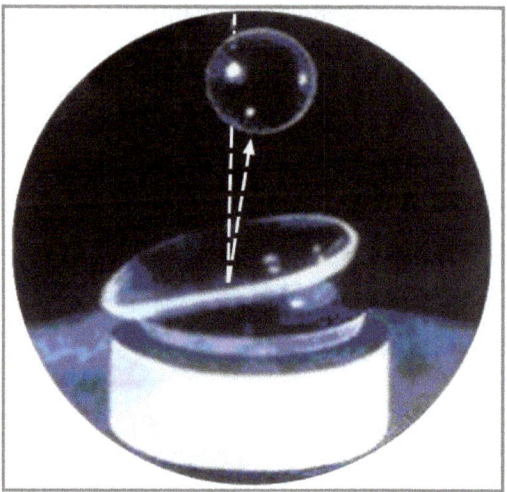

Fig. 12.4: Toughened lenses are impact resistance lenses. Normal glass lenses are processed to rearrange their molecular structure to withstand higher impact

withdrawn and cooled rapidly, usually by a jet of cold air. The sudden cooling creates a state of compression at the lens surface and a state of tension in the lens mass. This produces a compression tension coat, often referred to as the compression envelop. This improves the impact resistance which can be tested using drop ball test as shown in **Figure 12.4** to determine whether the lens has a certain minimum strength and cohesion under impact from a small hard object. In practice, thermally toughened glasses are also examined for the regularity of birefringence pattern for judgmental opinion of the impact resistance of the lens as shown in **Figure 12.5**. After the lenses have been manufactured, they are fitted into the frame or housing.

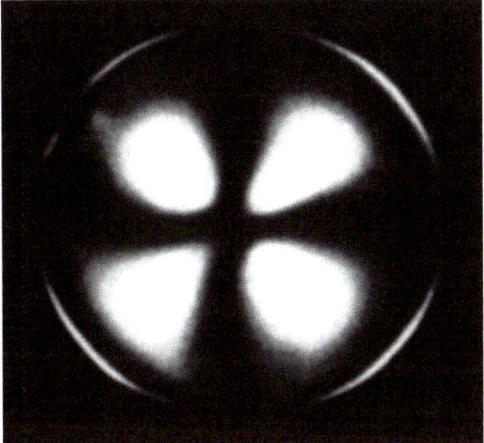

Fig. 12.5: Birefringence pattern of heat toughened glasses

Advantages
- Heat toughening is comparatively quick and cheap process.
- It does not need skilled labor.
- The equipment needed is inexpensive and requires little bench space.

Disadvantages
- Heat toughened lens will always be thicker than an untoughened lens of equivalent power.
- Prescription lenses over + 5.00 D are not ideal for toughening, as the bulk of glasses require prolonged heating which can cause warping, degrading the optical qualities. Lenses over – 5.00 D have poor impact resistance due to the relatively thin centre substance.
- Impact resistance is markedly reduced by scratches and other surface abrasions. Hence, they should be periodically inspected and replaced when distinct scratches are present.
- The heat toughening process has an adverse effect on the photo chromatic lenses. The lens does not lighten to its original transmission.

Chemically Toughened Glasses

In this process the lenses are first preheated and then lowered into a potassium nitrate solution at 470°C for 16 hours. The compression coat is produced by exchanging the larger potassium ions present in the solution for the smaller sodium ions present in the glass. As this treatment occurs on the surface of the glass only, it produces a very thin but very tough compression coat. For photo chromatic lens toughening, the solution normally used is 40% potassium nitrate and 60% sodium nitrate at a reduced temperature of 400°C. This process does not generally affect the photo chromatic action of the lenses.

Advantages
- Although, chemically toughened lenses are thinner than heat toughened lenses, they have been shown to possess a greater impact resistance.
- The toughening process takes the same time for all types of lenses.
- The temperature required for chemical toughening is lower than that used for the heat treatment of lenses; therefore, warping is not a problem.

Disadvantages
- Chemical toughening is an expensive process, as it requires equipments that must withstand the chemicals and the temperatures involved.
- It is difficult to determine whether the lens has been toughened, as there is neither a stress pattern nor a conventional method that will provide this information.
- It is not exactly suited for crown glasses. A special type of glass is needed for the best results which are more expensive.

When chemically or heat toughened glass lenses fracture, they usually show a radial fracture pattern, although concentric cracks can also occur. Therefore, only a few splinters of glass are produced and the fragments tend to stay in the spectacle frame.

Special Heat Toughened Safety Lenses

Special heat toughened lenses became widely available around 1970. The technology involved was developed by Chance Pilkington and is currently the property of Norville Optical Co. The lenses are heated in the same way as air-quenched lenses, but then cooled by immersion in oil. These lenses are somewhat thinner than the usual heat-toughened variety, and can be identified with a polarizing strain viewer. The strain pattern is obviously very different to that found in the conventional heat-toughened lens.

Plastics

There are different materials available in plastic material family:

CR_{39}

CR_{39} was introduced by the Columbia Chemical Division of the Pittsburg Plate Glass Company in 1941 and first became available as a spectacle lens material in 1950s. The word "CR" stands for Columbia Resin and it was the 39th batch or formula made by the laboratory. It is a thermosetting material and offers greater impact resistance. However, when the lens breaks, it produces sharper fragments. The scratches on the lens surface do not obviously affect the impact resistance.

Polycarbonate

Polycarbonate material was first produced in the late 1950, since then there has been a steady increase in its quality and use as it has been used to manufacture almost all safety devices as can be seen by **Figure 12.6 and 12.7**. Initially, the ophthalmic use of this material was restricted to industrial safety lenses as it was quite grey in appearance. But now polycarbonate lenses are readily available, not only as safety lenses, but also as high quality spectacle lenses for dress wear. Polycarbonate lenses are thermoplastic polymer that melts at a fairly low temperature and can be molded and remolded easily by a process of heating and cooling. When the strength of polycarbonate is compared to that of metals, the mechanical strength is fairly low, but it is very light and as a spectacle lens material they are very strong. Lenses can be produced by both molding and surfacing techniques with good quality impact resistant lenses. When hit polycarbonate crazes and the crazed areas that surrounds the point of impact can be seen easily by the way in which light is scattered through

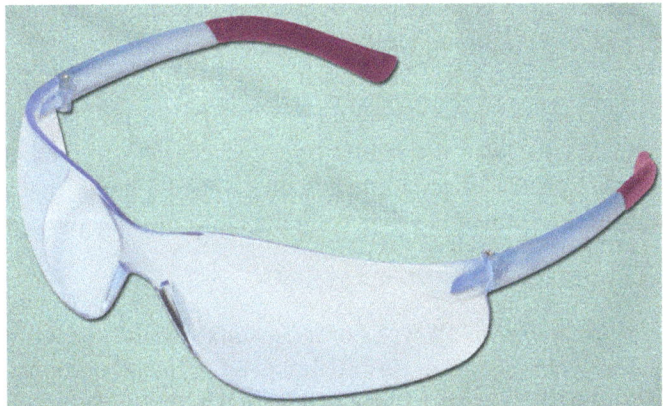

Fig. 12.6: Polycarbonate lenses

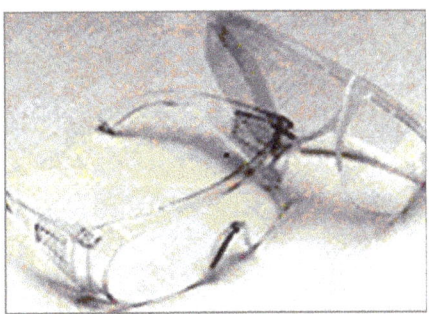
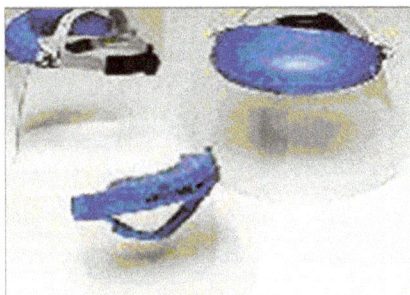

Fig. 12.7: Eye protectors and face shields

the lens. The amount of crazing produced is dependent on the time period of the load and the temperature of the material. When the temperature is low, the material crazes more readily and fractures by small high velocity particles occur at a low velocity. The surface of polycarbonate is fairly soft and scratches very easily. To overcome this problem, the usual practice is to hard coat the lens to protect its surface. Polycarbonate lenses are more difficult to glaze than CR39 lenses. Machines dedicated to this material are fitted with special edging wheels, as it is very difficult to cut using standard diamond-edging wheels.

Cellulose Acetate

This material has not been used to manufacture ophthalmic lenses as it is too soft to hold its shape accurately. However, it is used to make both frames and side-shields and to make covers to protect the surface of lenses.

Wire Gauze

Goggles made from wire gauze have a very good impact resistance, but are generally not accepted because they degrade the visual function and give no protection against splashes of molten metal, etc.

TESTING PROCEDURE FOR SAFETY LENSES

The lenses used as safety eyewear must be tested to establish whether they are suitable for the specific hazard for which they were designed. The important factors for testing parameters are given in the **Flowchart 12.3**.

Impact Resistance

The impact resistance of all types of lenses may be influenced when the surface has been abraded. The size and the speed of the missile or particle also influence the impact resistance of the lens. Larger particles hitting a lens cause it to bend, and so the fracture is initiated on the back surface. Smaller particles on the other hand do not cause the lens to bend upon impact, so the fracture is generally initiated on the front surface. The impact resistance also increases as the lens thickness increases. Increase in base curvature also increases the strength of the lens in both heat toughened and CR_{39} lenses.

Flowchart 12.3: Parameters for safety lens testing

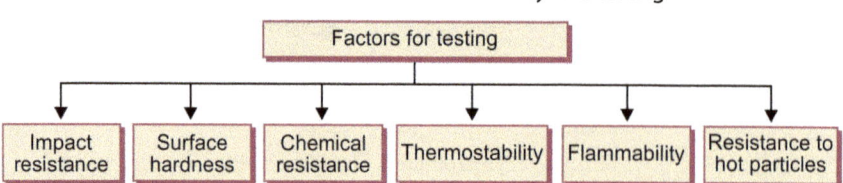

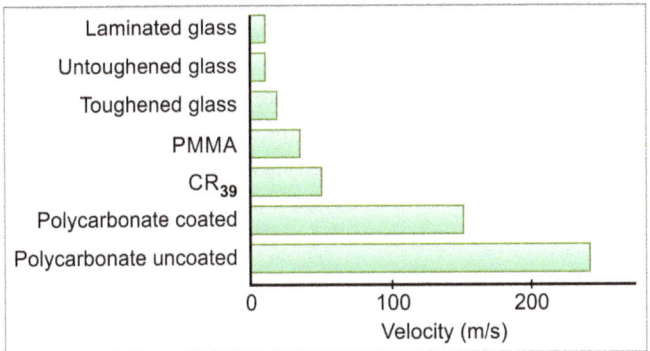

Fig. 12.8: Fracture velocity of a 3 mm thick sample of different lens materials when struck by a 6.5 mm diameter steel ball

The type of material used for safety eyewear gives an indication of the mean fracture velocity that can be tolerated. **Figure 12.8** shows the fracture velocity for some of the materials available. The samples were all of the same thickness and were struck by a 6.5 mm steel ball. Polycarbonate offers the greatest fracture resistance of all the lens material.

Surface Hardness

There have been many efforts to study the problems associated with surface abrasion. However, there are distinct advantages in coating plastic lenses, particularly polycarbonate, which is soft thermoplastic. A thinly coated polycarbonate lens is superior to an uncoated CR_{39} lenses.

Chemical Resistance

Glasses are more resistant to most chemicals. Plastics, however, may show crazing and surface clouding with some strong chemical solutions. CR_{39} has good chemical resistance, and is frequently used for chemical visors and box goggle windows.

Thermostability

Polycarbonate and PMMA are prone to distortion more readily than glasses.

Flammability

All the plastic materials are flammable. However, as their ignition temperatures are high, they are considered safe for use.

Resistance to Hot Particles

Figure 12.9 shows glass material is pitted more than the CR 39 material when exposed to hot particles which makes it more vulnerable. Eye protectors must be able to withstand hot particles impinging upon them, as can occur in such processes as grinding or welding. A glass surface is very easily pitted by these particles, as they fuse with the surface. Whereas, plastics do not pit easily. This could be due to the elasticity of the surface when heated by the particle.

Table 12.1 gives the complete synopsis of different materials used as safety lenses against different testing parameters.

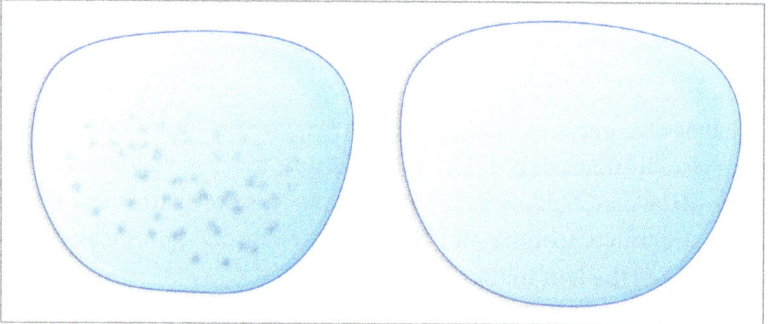

Fig. 12.9: Resistance to hot particles by a glass lens (left) and a CR_{39} (right) lens. After equal exposure to spatter from an arc welder the glass lens is considerably more pitted than the CR_{39} lenses

Table 12.1: A Comparison of the major properties

Material	Impact resistance		Hardness	Chemical resistance	Thermostability	Fracture pattern particles	Resistance to hot	Weight
	Large Missile	Small Missile						
Glass								
Heat toughened	Good	Good	Good	Very good	Very good	Fair	Poor	Heaviest
Chemically toughened	Good	Poor	Good	Very good	Very good	Fair	Poor	Heavy
Laminated	Fair	Fair	Good	Good	Fair	Poor	Poor	Heavy
Plastics								
PMMA	Fair	Fair	Poor	Good	Fair	Good	Very good	Light
CR39	Good	Good	Fair	Good	Good	Fair	Good	Light
Polycarbonate (coated)	Very good	Very good	Poor	Fair	Good	Very good	Good	Light

TYPES OF LENS HOUSING

The lens housing may be made of metal or plastics. Nickel alloy is usually used to make metal housing and polycarbonate, polyamide, cellulose acetate, etc can be used for plastic lens housing. These materials may be used to manufacture:
- Spectacle frames
- Goggles
- Face shields
- Helmets

Spectacle Frames

Cellulose acetate, polyamide, polycarbonate and many other kinds of plastics can be used to make plastic spectacle frames. They can also be made from metal wire also, but these frames have been shown to cause more damage upon impact than a plastic frame. Side shield spectacle frames as shown in **Figure 12.10** are very good as eye-protectors. But these side shields must not restrict the wearers field of vision and hence they should be made of transparent material that does not discolor with age. Injection molded side shields with polycarbonate materials are best, as their shape does not alter.

Goggles

The goggles can be made either cup type or box type for eye protection purpose. The cup type may be used to provide protection against molten metal, flying particles, dust etc. Box type goggles give a good fit around the brows and cheeks. They can also be worn over prescription spectacles.

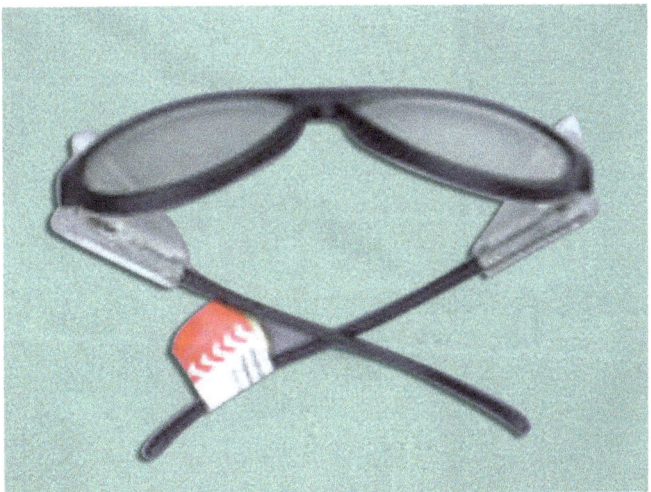

Fig. 12.10: Side shield spectacle frame

Face Shields

Face shields (**Fig. 12.11**) are usually head band supported visors that cover the face and neck. They are used to provide protection from flying particles, molten metal and chemical splashes and can easily be worn over prescription spectacles, if required. They provide excellent field of view. Face shields are usually made either from polycarbonate or cellulose acetate.

Helmets

Helmets are commonly worn during welding. They provide protection of the face and neck from intense radiation and spatter. The filters can also be attached which can also be so designed that it can be flipped up to expose.

■ REGULATIONS AND STANDARDS RELATING TO EYE PROTECTION

The British and European Standards for eye protectors BS EN 166:2000 Personal Eye Protection Specification is at the heart of the strategy for eye protectors, but other standards like USA .... ANSI Z 87.1, Canada .... CSA Z 94 etc are also linked to it.

BS EN 165 – specifies personal eye protection vocabulary.

BS EN 166 – personal eye protection – specification.

BS EN 167 –specifies optical test methods.

BS EN 168 – specifies non optical test methods.

BS EN 169 – specifies tints for welding protection and similar operation.

BS EN 170 – specifies for UV filters.

BS EN 171 – specifies for IR filters.

BS EN 172 – specifies for sun glare filters.

BS EN 175 – specifies for ski-goggles.

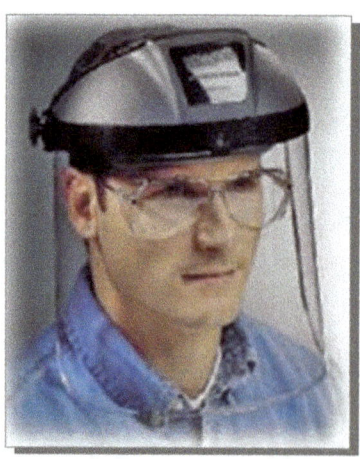

Fig. 12.11: Face shields

BS EN 207 – specifies for filters and eye protectors against laser radiation.
BS EN 208 –Laser adjustment eye protectors.
BS 7930 – 1:1998 – Eye protectors for racket sports. Part 1 Squash.
BS 4110 – Eye visors for vehicle users.

Most BS EN standards use the specifications in BS EN 166. The old BS standards tend to use different specifications. BS EN 166 was first issued in 1994 and superseded BS 2092. It is now more than 10years old and was last amended in 2002. The standards there in are the most important to an optometrist.

A typical safety spectacle has the following lens markings:

5- 3.1 "AOS" 1 F

The first digit, i.e., 5 is the code number. This specifies the wavelength of the radiation that the filter offers protection against **(Table 12.2)**.

The second 3.1 is the shade number. The shade number signifies the tint density. The shade number ranges from 1.1 to 4.1. Welding filters are often specified with shade number only. 1.1 corresponds to the light transmission factor of 80% which is maximum permissible tint for night driving. 3 correspond to an light transmission factor of 17.8 to 8.5%—the maximum permissible tint for driving in day light.

The optical class is signified by the number 1 **(Table 12.3)**. The optical class indicates the measure of optical tolerance to which the lenses have been manufactured. Prescription safety eyewear needs to be checked to the same standards as normal spectacles and can be marked only 1 or 2. Class 3 is only to be used in eye protectors that are not to be used for long use.

Table 12.2: 1 BS EN 166 Code numbers for filters

Filter code no.	Filter property
No code no.	Welding filters
2.	UV filter where colour recognition may be affected
3.	UV filter with good colour recognition
4.	IR filter
5.	Sun glare filter without IR specification
6.	Sun glare filter with IR specification

Table 12.3: BS EN 166 – Optical Class – Tolerances

Number	Sph and cyl	Horizontal prism	Vertical prism
1.	+, – 0.06D	0.75 deg out 0.25 deg in	0.25 deg up and down
2.	+, – 0.12D	1.0 deg out 0.25 deg in	0.25 deg up and down
3.	+ 0.12D-0.25D	1.00 deg out 0.25 deg in	0.25 deg up and down

Table 12.4: Grades of impact resistance BS EN 166

Symbol	Level of impact resistance	Test ball speed	Best material can achieve
F	Low energy	45 m/s	All types
B	Medium energy	120 m/s	Goggles and face shields.
A	High energy	190 m/s	Face shields
S	Increased robustness	—	Toughened glass

F on the oculars signifies the impact resistance **(Table 12.4)**. There are two tests for increased robustness:

1. The oculars have to withstand the impact of a 22 mm diameter steel ball weighing 43 g traveling at 5.1 m/s.
2. The eye protectors must withstand the impact of a 6 mm diameter steel ball weighing 0.86 g traveling at 12 m/s.

The letter 'T', for example, FT after impact resistance shows that the eye protectors will be effective at higher temperature also.

Multiple Choice Questions (MCQs)

1. The common mechanical hazards associated with eyes is:
    a. Cataract
    b. Sub-conjunctival hemorrhage
    c. Black eye
    d. All of the above

2. Which of the following ocular hazard is associated with visible light of the electromagnetic spectrum?
    a. Retinal burns
    b. Pterygium
    c. Pingeculae
    d. Corneal abrasion

Answers

1. d   2. a

Chapter 13

Surface Treatments

There are various kinds of surface treatments that are applied on either side of the spectacle lenses. In addition to anti-reflection coating which has already been discussed separately, many other types of surface treatments are done to enhance optical and/or physical properties of the lens. Optical properties can be enhanced by tinting, UV coating and mirror coating and the physical enhancements can be achieved by hard coating, hydrophobic coating, anti-mist coating and anti-fog coating as shown in **Figure 13.1**.

■ HARD COATING

Plastic lenses are extremely light in weight and hence very comfortable to wear but their relatively soft surfaces make them prone to scratches. To minimize the possibility of scratches plastic lenses can be coated from both sides with a hard protective coating. The 2 micron thick hard coating makes the lens surface more resistant to scratches and therefore increases the durability of the lenses. Hard coating provides following advantages:
- It makes the lens more resistant to scratches
- It ensures greater durability

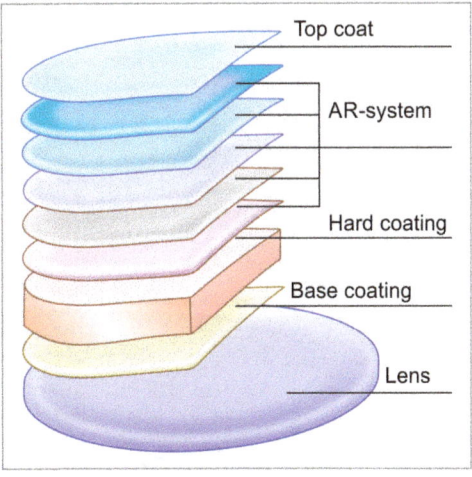

Fig. 13.1: Different layers of coating on a lens

- It ensures easier lens cleaning
- The visual performance of the lens is enhanced for longer time.

There are several ways of applying hard coatings. Spin coating and Dip coating are most popular among them. Hard coating can also be applied by vacuum deposition process which is usually done when it is combined with Anti-reflection coating also. Hard coatings are usually applied using various types of varnishes These varnishes are available in different indices to suit the different indices of lens substrates. Varnishes having index of 1.50 is categorized as low index varnish and 1.52 is mid index varnish and 1.58 to 1.60 indices are usually classified as high index varnishes. The higher the refractive index of the lens substrate, the higher index varnish is needed. The important benefits of such matched coating is its high quality adhesive strength and avoidance of annoying interference resulting in cosmetically attractive lenses in every respect. The thickness of coating layer is regulated by the speed at which the lenses are immersed and removed from the lacquer and also by it viscosity. Viscosity of lacquer is very critical to maintain for which a constant temperature of 18 degree celcius must be maintained. Once the lacquer is applied to lenses, the lenses are cured either by UV rays or by thermal curing. However, before putting the lenses into the lacquer, they are vigorously cleaned and etched. Etching ensures strong adhesion. Polycarbonate lens material also needs a layer of primer coat before applying hard coating. Hard coating may be tintable or non-tintable. Non-tintable coating offers more scratch resistance.

HYDROPHOBIC COATING

Hydrophobic coating as shown in **Figure 13.2**, is a very thin layer of a few molecules applied on top of anti-reflection coating as a protective layer. It

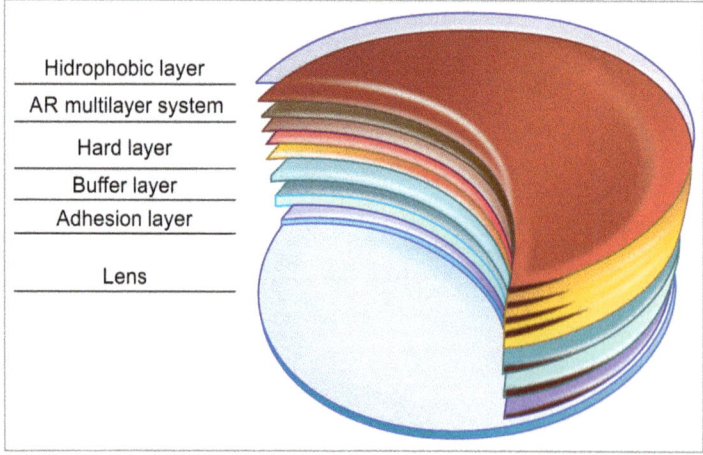

Fig. 13.2: Top layer coating is hydrophobic coating

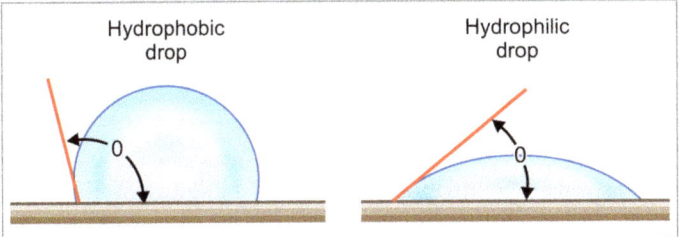

Fig. 13.3: High surface wetting angle

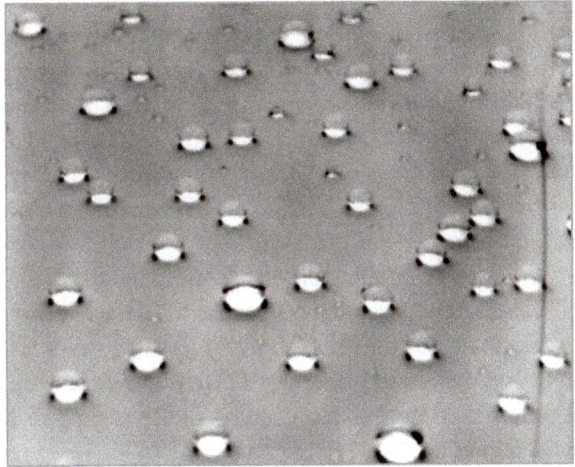

Fig. 13.4: Water droplets on a hydrophobic coating

repels water by an electrochemical molecule repulsion, thus prevents water marks and also grease marks, which makes the lens cleaning an easier process. Since it is very thin, it does not interfere with the optics of Anti-reflection coating. The basic principle is to create a high surface wetting angle as shown in **Figure 13.3**, which allows the water or oil to run off rather than wetting and then drying on the surface **(Fig. 13.4)**. It can be applied simply by dipping process. Baking after dipping enhances the life. It can also be applied in the vacuum chamber as the final stage of the multi-layer anti-reflection coating process.

▌ ANTI-FOG COATING

The potential for eye injuries in sports and battlefield has increased over the years. Fogging of spectacle lenses can occur from a combination of body heat and environmental factors which can result in blur vision from sweat beads streaming down the lenses. A film of anti-fog coating can be applied on the back surface of the lens which is compatible with hard coating to protect the lens from being fogged. A good anti-fogging treatment has not only initial anti-fogging properties but also good anti-fogging retainability. At times anti-fogging lens cleaning solutions have been used in the form of sprays, the effect of the same has yet to be studied.

ANTI-MIST COATING

The same reason can be attributed to anti-mist coating on the lens surface. The property to prevent the formation of mist behind the lens is an important feature.

TOUGHENING GLASS LENSES

Spectacle glass lenses can be strengthened by toughening process. The finished lens is heated to its softening point and is followed by rapid cooling, either by a stream of cold compressed air directed at the surfaces or by submerging the lens in oil. This results in greater compressive strength in the glass since outer region of the lens material cools more rapidly than the interior, which remains hotter and more fluid for some time. When the interior finally cools, it contracts and exerts tension on the rigid outer surface to produce an envelope that encloses the interior under great tensile stress. Toughened glasses are far more durable and more resistant to scratches because of increased surface hardness. When they break, they shatter into relatively harmless cubes of glasses. In practice, thermally toughened glasses can be examined for the regularity of birefringence pattern for judgmental opinion of the impact resistance of the lens as shown in **Figure 13.5**.

Glasses can also be toughened by a chemical process, in which a compressive envelop, is produced by ion exchange as a result of hot dip of the finished lens into a salt bath. Chemically toughened lenses are stronger than air-quenched toughened lenses.

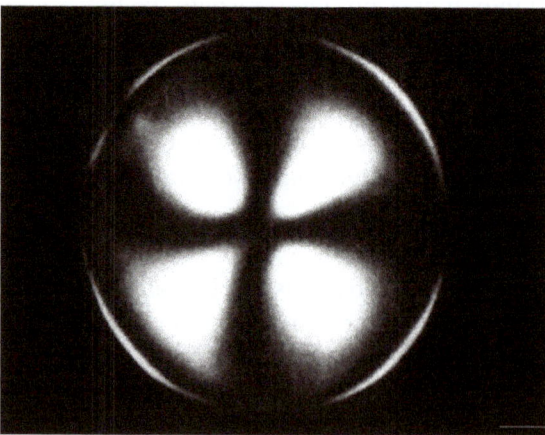

Fig. 13.5: Birefringence pattern of thermally toughened lens

SURFACE TINTING OF LENSES

Tints are simply the methods of absorbing lights so that transmission is reduced. If all wavelengths of light are equally absorbed, then a neutral grey is produced. If the absorption is different for different wavelengths, then the tint has a particular color. Tinting resin lenses are relatively simple procedure. The lenses are placed in a suitable bath of hot color dye for an appropriate length of time. Excess darkness can be reduced and light color can be made darker. Full color and graduated colors are all possible **(Fig. 13.6)**. Glasses can also be coated by vacuum process **(Fig. 13.7)** which has a unique advantage of uniform tint throughout the lens surface which is otherwise not possible in glass lenses.

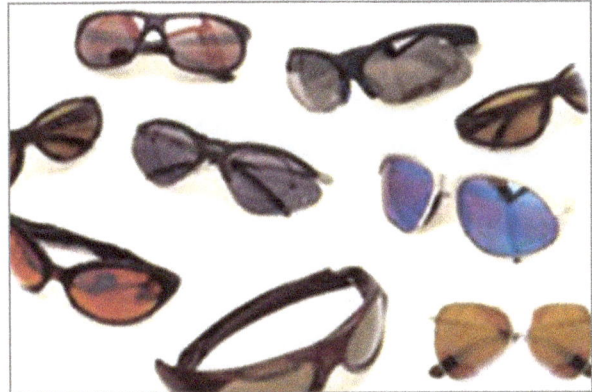

Fig. 13.6: Varieties of tinted lenses

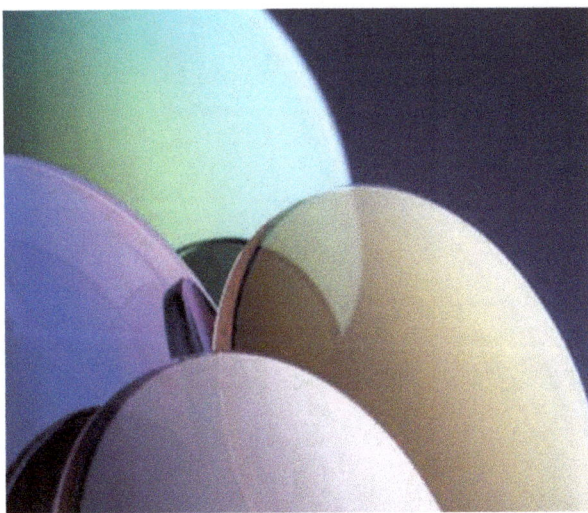

Fig. 13.7: Mirror coating

Multiple Choice Questions (MCQs)

1. Which of the following surface treatment is not applied to spectacle lenses with an objective to enhance the optical properties of the lenses:
   a. Tinting
   b. Hydrophobic coating
   c. Mirror coating
   d. Anti-reflective coating

2. Which of the following surface treatment is applied to spectacle lenses for physical enhancements?
   a. Hard coating
   b. Hydrophobic coating
   c. Anti-mist coating
   d. All of the above

Answers

1. b   2. d

Chapter 14

Sports Lenses

The world in which we live has become more diverse and varied than it was before. Increasing complexities and ever increasing demands have changed lots of old philosophies. Today the concept of "one size for all" philosophy has no more importance. Both in the workplace and at leisure, things have changed. With so much of changes clear, comfortable and good vision in variety of situations also necessitate the need for specialized products and services for specialized occupation. The increasing competition in all spheres has further added to the fact that one can not take the chance any more. One mistake means the entire career is over.

Sports, today is one of the largest industries where more than 50% population of the world is engaged professionally or otherwise. Eyesight is extremely important in sports, especially when it comes to skiing and ice hockey. In dazzling light of the high mountains, where the sun's rays are multiplied by reflections and fresh snow, in thick snowdrifts and incident fog, visual perception is seriously limited. The complex movements are continuously coordinated, controlled and corrected by means of visual inspection.

Compared to the rest of the body, the high energy consumption of the eye frequently results in faster fatigue. Moreover, the eye has to adapt not only to the very strong light of the wave spectrum visible to human eyes, but also needs to be protected for longer use. At high altitudes, filter function is reduced. Protection is also diminished since ozone layer is thinner as you go higher. Ultraviolet light has very high damaging effect on our eyes. The omnipresent Infrared rays above 800 nm carry thermal effect on the eyes. In the enclosed spaces light intensity is less than the open spaces. There may be possibility that regular glasses, fitted in a normal or dress wear every day frame **(Fig. 14.1)** may not give the adequate vision that a player is needed. At times he may be tired of not being able to accurately read the green and

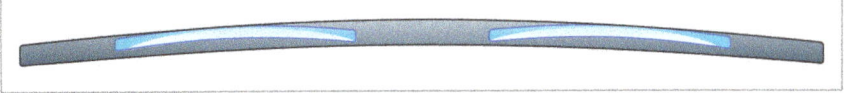

Fig. 14.1: Everyday frame

sink that putt. The glare coming off the water surface on sunny days while fishing or boating creates visual noise and wind making their eyes dry when they really get moving on the new mountain bike. Wind, flying dirt and debris can cause itchy and irritated eyes. So protection is an important factor while dispensing lenses to the player. Each sport requires some sort of protection from high speed projectiles to play safely and comfortably. Besides protection, enhancing vision for superior performance is also very critical in sports.

The big advantage of an optical appliance is that they allow the eyes to be protected. A well designed sports specific frame is usually wrapping around the face **(Fig. 14.2)** following the facial anatomy, protecting against light, particles and insects from the sides and above and also shielding the eyes from pollen and wind, in contrast to everyday frame which are fairly flat across the front.

With the right choice of lens, complete UV protection can be given and by removing blue and UV light, contrast enhancement can be achieved which is directly related to increased sporting performance. However, use of wrap around frames for prescription means that standard calculations are no longer valid because of the way in which the frames wraps around the eyes and cause:
- Change in dioptric power
- Unwanted prismatic effects
- Oblique astigmatism.

The lens tilt also leads to induced decent ration. In addition, the high base curve lens leads to impaired optical properties in the periphery and one of the essentials of a sports spectacle is to enhance peripheral vision.

However, the use of wrap around frames for prescription means that standard calculations that are commonly used to design spectacle lenses are not valid because of the way in which the frames wrap around the face and fits in front of the eyes and it causes unusual effect as shown in **Flowchart 14.1**.

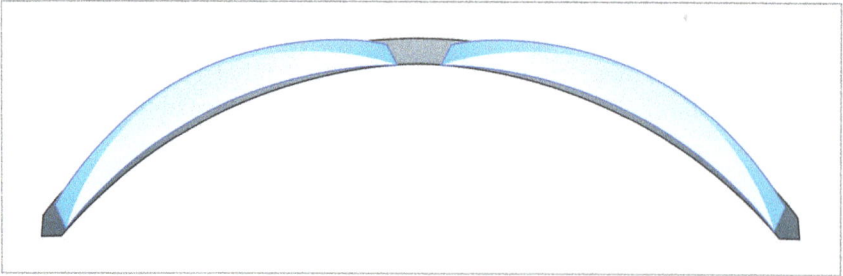

Fig. 14.2: Sports frame

Flowchart 14.1: Undesirable effects of sports frames

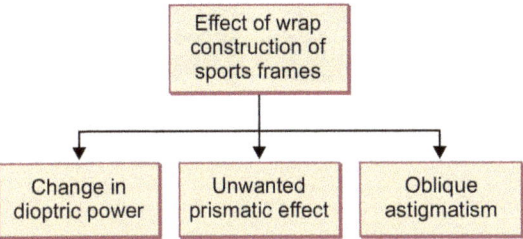

The lens tilt also leads to induced decentration. It happens because the visual axis of the frame doesn't correspond to the optical axis of the lens. The new configuration of the fitting implies that the wearer is now looking through the lens on a different optical axis corresponding to the wrapped positioning. It induces unwanted prism, oblique astigmatism and blur and also leads to impaired optical properties in the lens periphery and one of the essentials of sports spectacle lens is to enhance the peripheral vision. This necessitates the need for compensatory lens prescription to calculate the new lens prescription on X and Y axis so that result can be improved on Z-axis as shown in **Figure 14.3** that will maintain visual clarity at all angles of view even at the edge of the lens.

The solution to this is specially designed spectacle lenses which are customized to meet most prescription needs in terms of factors that are shown in **Flowchart 14.2** with the aim of fitting the lenses directly into the frame.

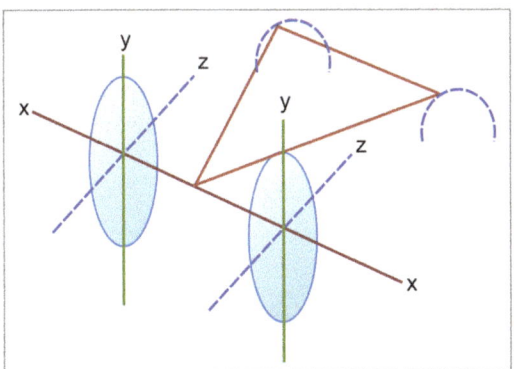

Fig. 14.3: XYZ optics maintains the visual clarity at all angles of view even at the edge of the lens

Flowchart 14.2: Three important factors

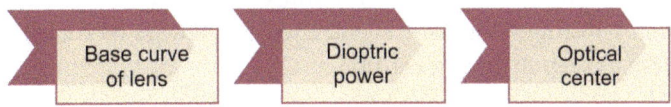

Flowchart 14.3:: Dispensing measurements to consider while dispensing sports lenses

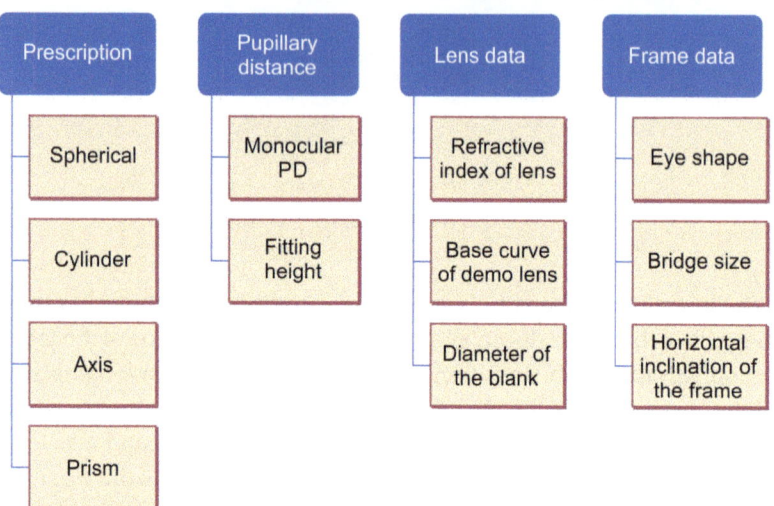

This necessitates recalculations of lens power that compensates for above errors, the lenses so prepared are commonly known as sports lenses. The dispensing of sports lenses requires that the dispensing measurements as shown in **Flowchart 14.3** should be taken into considerations while dispensing sports lenses:

Based upon above information, the sports lens software calculates an aberrationally corrected dioptric lens power and optimizes the centering data to provide wider peripheral field of view and clear vision through the lens size.

The solution to this is especially designed spectacle lenses which are individually manufactured to meet most prescription needs in terms of the following with the aim of fitting the lenses directly into the frames:
- The base curve
- The dioptric power
- The cent ration.

■ HORIZONTAL INCLINATION

Horizontal inclination is measured by drawing a tangent to the optical centre of the lens and noting the angle it makes with the front plane of the frame. As it is clear from **Figure 14.4** that the visual axis of a sports frame does not correspond to the optical axis of the lens and this is really the reason why we need to make compensations for sports lens dispensing. There will be some adjustments in the dioptric power and/or cylinder with some deviation in axis and unwanted prismatic effect. There will always be some decent ration required as seen in the **Figure 14.5**.

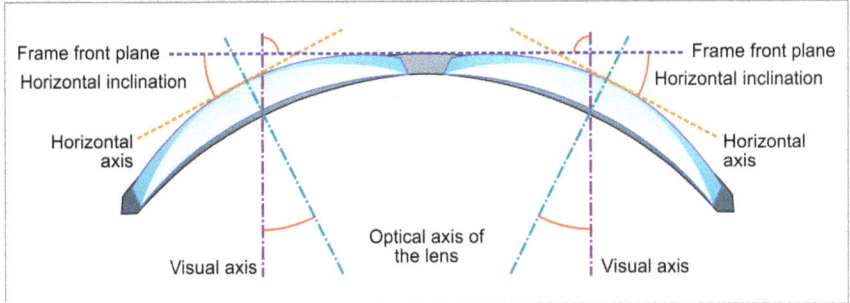

Fig. 14.4: Horizontal inclination

		Sph.	Cyl.	A.	Pr.
Prescription		+ 3.25	+ 0.75	155	....
Horizontal inclination, frame not in wear 29°		+ 2.50	+ 1.25	168°	1.21
Horizontal inclination, with a small head, frame in wear 29°		+ 2.75	+ 1.00	166°	1.04
Horizontal inclination, with a large head, frame in wear 19°		+ 3.00	+ 1.00	161°	....

Fig. 14.5: Change of dioptric power in ratio changing horizontal inclination

Measuring Horizontal Inclination

While measuring the horizontal inclination, the frame must be on the head of the athlete because the spreading of the sides as the frame passes over the temples tends to decrease the horizontal inclination **(Fig. 14.6)** and the measurements must be made in this situation. It is not sufficient to take these measurements on the frame on its own. The following step has to be followed to take the measurement of horizontal inclination:

- Determine the geometric center: Mark the geometric center on the demo lens with vertical line using boxed lens system. The boxing system is based upon the idea of drawing an imaginary box around a lens shape with the box's sides tangent to the outer most edges of the shape. The system uses the sides of the boxes as reference points for the standard system of measurements **(Fig. 14.7)**.

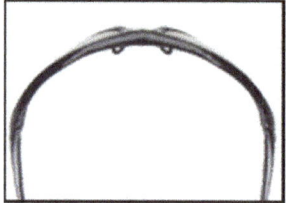 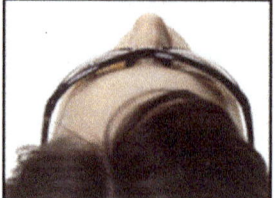 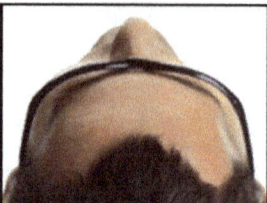

Horizontal inclination, frame not in wear 29°   Horizontal inclination, with a small head, frame in wear 26°   Horizontal inclination, with a large head, frame in wear 19°

Fig. 14.6: Changes in horizontal inclination as noted with change in facial width

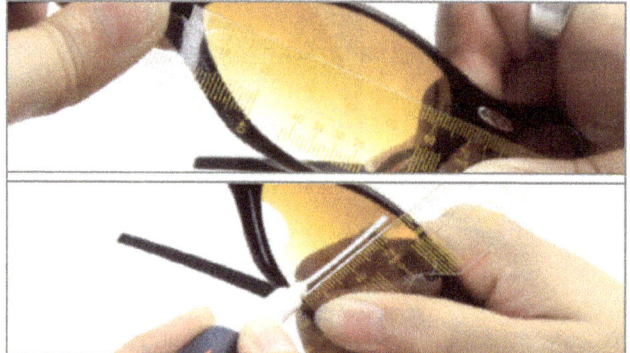

Fig. 14.7: Step no. 1

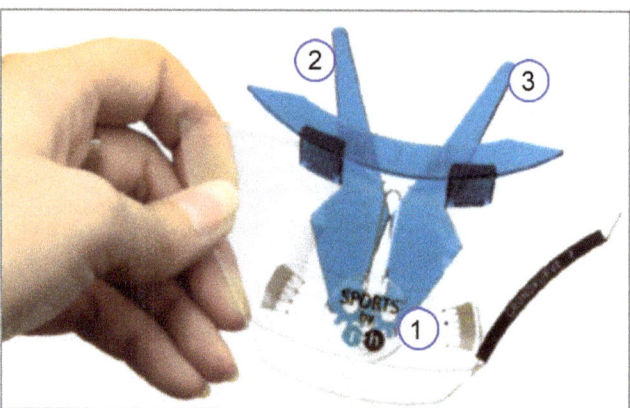

Fig. 14.8: Step no. 2

- Prepare the measuring aid: The easier way to take the measurement is to prepare the measuring aid as shown in the **Figure 14.8**, setting knob (1) back, measuring arms (2) and (3) closed.
- Place the measurement aid on the frame: Now place the measuring aid onto the frame. When you place the aid, the measuring arms open. Make sure

that the guide bar (4) is apposed to the upper edge of the frame and the mid marking of the guide bar accords with the frame mid point **(Fig. 14.9)**.
- Adjust horizontal inclination: Adjust the measuring arms (2) and (3) by moving the setting knob forward. When the measuring arms rest on the lens vertical marking they are at the correct angle **(Fig. 14.10)**.
- Read the horizontal inclination: Read the angle at the point where the measuring arm accords with the scale **(Fig. 14.11)**.

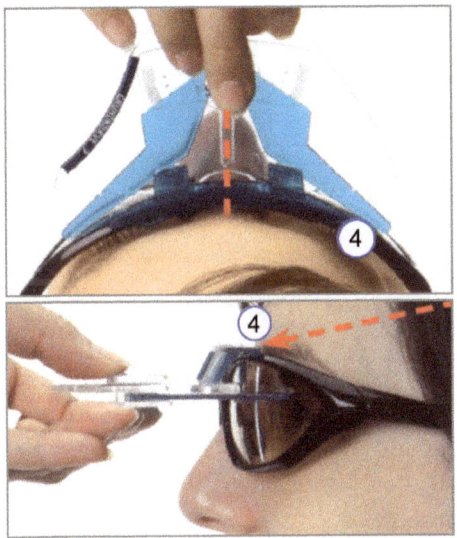

Fig. 14.9: Step no. 3

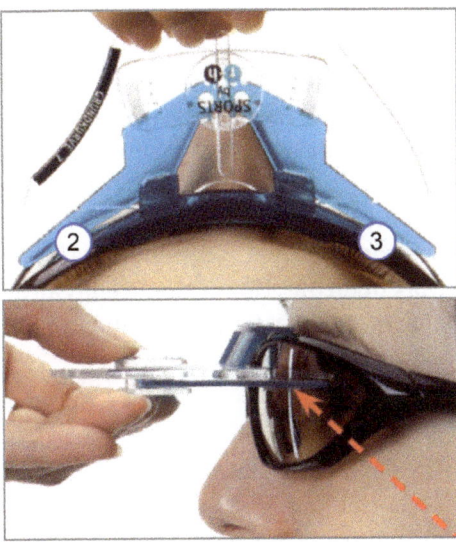

Fig. 14.10: Step no. 4

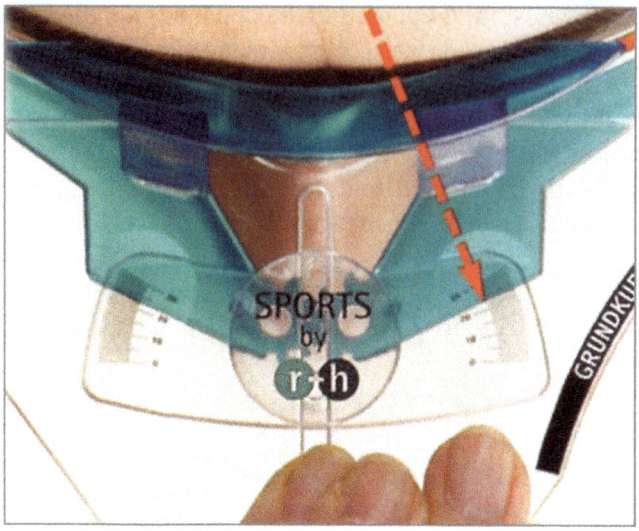

Fig. 14.11: Step no. 5

■ FEATURES OF SPORT LENSES

In sports vision is maximized by the correct use of lenses and trauma is avoided by the correct use of lens material. Everything that is being to protect and enhance vision has a bearing on safety. This sums up the following features of a good sports lens:

Impact Resistant Material

Sport is the commonest cause of severe eye injuries in the world today. People who get eye injuries in sports were not wearing eye protection. Over the last 10 years, the popularity of sports has increased enormously. There are a few standards enforced by the state. The purpose of standards is to make sure that the practitioners know what is available to ensure required protection in each sport. Unless the standards are available, advice and knowledge will inevitably vary from one practitioner to another. In such cases some athletes may get wrong advice. The need for protection of eyes in sports is evident and the ruling bodies will have to work upon this. However, currently all the sports lenses are made of polycarbonate or trivex material. It is difficult to justify anything less. Due to cost factor some may use CR_{39} lenses also.

Ultraviolet Protection

The pathogenesis of ocular disease due to UV is well understood. Sports lenses reduce the amount of shorter wavelength non-ionizing radiations reaching the retina and also useful to provide protection to the ocular adnexa.

Anti-reflection Coating

In terms of light transmission, anti-reflection coatings are applied on both the surface of the lens. These coatings increase light transmission from 92% to up to 99%. The increase in visual information must improve contrast sensitivity and will particularly important in poor light.

Water Repellent

Anti-reflection coating can be made water repellent. This is very important as visual demands in sports can not be compromised.

Anti-mist Coating

The same reason can be attributed to anti-mist coating on the lens surface. The property to prevent the formation of mist behind the lens is an important feature.

Scratch Resistant Hard Coating

Loss of vision due to scratches can not be accepted in sports lenses. They must be treated with hard scratch resistant coating which is not compromising as far as light transmission is concerned.

Optically Compensated Lenses

High curve lenses are designed to be fitted in wrap around sports frames. The new configuration of the fitting implies that the wearer is now looking through the lens on a different optical axis corresponding to the wrapped positioning. The effect is seen as induced prismatic error, power error and oblique astigmatism which require a compensatory lens power. The greater the degree of the wrap angle of the frame, the greater amount of compensating lens power will be required.

■ TINTS AND COLORS IN SPORTS LENSES

When things go wrong with the visual system, it may have a profound effect on the everything we do. For some people changing the color of their world may produce interesting and surprising results. The usefulness of color and tints has already been seen in hospital eye screening as clinically significant in cases like albinism, aniridia, ARMD, cataracts and aphakia. Light sensitive people have been using dark tints comfortably to protect their eyes from intense light. Given the potential of tints to relieve symptoms and prevent diseases, it has been found necessary to have a standard method to test the color preference in general practice. Research in the field of sportvision has already established the merits of Eyebright Test. The tint that is being preferred in the aforesaid test is the summation of psychological as well as its physical properties. It may not be duplicated in the spectacle, but is the guide to the practitioner to decide final prescription on clinical judgments based on their optical principle and degree of light sensitivity. Commonly LT 80% is the first choice for indoors and LT 20% for sun. The important thing is that tints are not occupation specific, they are person specific. Hence, the results of the Eyebright test are very important. However, considering the environmental conditions needed for different sports a general guideline can be worked upon what tints have been seen to be most effective in different sports:

- *Orange:* In normal use, orange is the essence of brown, so a tint diagnosis of orange would translate to brown tint. Using clinical judgments, this would be given indoors or outdoors at appropriate transmission level. Orange is the most commonly used tint for clay shooting. They are good to enhance visual performance and comfort, shooting sports require lenses that increase visibility of targets, dampen backgrounds, ease eyestrain and fatigue, and provide protection from harmful sunlight. Hunters and other target shooters also benefit from orange tint.
- *Green:* The diagnostic green is not usually prescribed unless for a specific purpose. It makes a very good sunglass tint, because of its contrast enhancing properties and good UV absorption. Green is also good IR absorber. Golfers rely heavily on green filter to distinguish the ball from green.
- *Blue:* In particularly light sensitive subjects, the light scattering effect of blue is outweighed by the relief they get from the elimination of peak sensitivity wavelengths of yellow and orange. However, blue is absolutely contraindicated for outdoor use because of the danger of high energy blue light intensified by the brilliance of sun.
- *Yellow*: A yellow filter increases the contrast between that color and surrounding colors, and concentrates light in the area of the spectrum to which the eye is most sensitive. If an individual is already light sensitive then the experience is heightened looking through a yellow or orange filter. Contrast is also enhanced by its absorption of blue and UV, which makes it effective for night driving against oncoming headlights and in fog. In fading light , sports players may appreciate the effect on contrast. It is not suitable as a sun spectacle because of glare and toxic effect of light at peak spectral sensitivity. Hunters, pilots, shooters and tennis players find them helpful for this purpose.
- *Pink:* Pink is the color second least chosen but is an indication of low light sensitivity. Migraine sufferors favor this color for indoor. For outdoor sun protection, second choice would be brown and green. It helps block blue light thereby improving contrast and offers high contrast and are very soothing to the eyes. It also improves road visibility. Many people feel that

pink lenses are more comfortable for long periods of time than other lenses. They are great for computer users to reduce eyestrain and glare.
- *Fuchsia:* This is often confused with pink but is actually from the shorter wavelength end of the spectrum and is the part of the family of violet and purple and is least chosen color . Like blue it is favored by light sensitive because of its tendency to absorb all the higher wavelengths, but is too dark even for the most light sensitive patients. Its contrast enhancing properties are likely to be poor.
- *Grey:* Grey is a neutral density filter which does not distort color. Gray is the general purpose tint because it tames bright sunlight. It is likely to be favored by the light sensitive and those who can not tolerate color distortion or whose job requires accurate color discrimination as it absorbs equally over the whole spectrum. It is not the contrast enhancer and is the natural alternative to green in photo chromatic lenses. It is cosmetically good for indoor use to reduce glare from fluorescent lamps, VDU and television screen.
- *Polaroid lens*: Polaroid lenses work similar to a Venetian blind by only letting in light at certain angles. Without the sun's glare, objects become more distinct and are seen in their true colors. Reduced glare off water, roads, and other objects make the polarized lens a favorite for water sports, fishing, cycling and driving. The additional density of silver mirror front complimented by back anti-reflection coating can be a great for sunny day fishing. Polarized lenses may be appropriate for the recreational skier, but as polarized lenses eliminate almost all reflected glare, they might pose a hazard for the professional or more accomplished participant. These athletes must be able to spot and respond quickly to ice and water patches. These would be all but invisible with polarized lenses. A more effective choice would be a mirror coating. Mirrors limit glare without eliminating it, offering the contrasts needed. Mirrors also add to the overall absorption of the lens. The denser the mirror coat, the more the absorption.
- *Photo chromatic lenses:* In changeable weather conditions or in sport where you are moving from areas of bright light to shade (for example golf and cycling) photochromic lenses are useful. These lenses darken in bright light and become paler in less intense light conditions.

Mirror Coating in Sports Lens

Mirror coatings on the lens not only look good but also provide a variety of visual benefits. Mirror lenses have changed considerably in recent years as technology has made it possible to create nearly limitless mirror colors and densities. Today's mirrors offer a broad range of possibilities and improved optical performance for both prescription and non-prescription wearers. Sure, colored mirror coatings are prevalent on sports lenses, and flash coatings have found a fashion home on Rx. lenses, but there are also some medical conditions that benefit from mirror coatings. The flash mirror coating creates a dynamic effect because the lenses appear to change color depending on how the light hits them. The latest trend in mirror coated lenses is the lightly visible "clear" mirror. Mirror coatings have become hugely popular on sports performance sun wear. Their color and density are matched with the base lens colors tint to enhance the wearers visual comfort and performance. You'll find mirror tints specifically designed for water sports, land sports, snow sports, general sports, and bright sun. Light transmission in a mirror coated lens is reduced because of the high percentage of light being reflected. Mirrors reflect more infrared and ultra-violet than they do visible light, which will benefit patients bothered by glare or affected by dry eye.

The simple rule to select the suitable color is by developing contrast absorptions which is possible by determining the color of the object being focused on and matching the color of the lens to the object. The color of that item will become more vivid. The other option is to use a lens color that matches the background. That color will be enhanced, so the object being located will be more apparent in its difference. In short we can analyse the application of tints in various sports as under:

Golf	:	Green tint
Tennis	:	Yellow tint
Clay pigeon	:	Orange tint
Target shooting	:	Yellow tint
Fishing, Sailing	:	Polaroid lens.
Skiing	:	Polaroid lens, orange or yellow tint.
Scuba diving	:	Blue, or bluey grey tint
Table tennis	:	Yellow tint
Cricket	:	Photo chromatic or orange, red tint.
Driving	:	Polaroid lens, or brown tint
Cycling, skating	:	Brown tint
Swimming	:	Blue, or bluey grey tint

■ PRESBYOPIA AND SPORTS LENS

Presbyopia does not stop people playing sports. The important fact is that presbyopia has an ongoing effect on your eyes, so your corrective lens prescription may need to be changed over time, as a result. So sports progressives are very important.

With most sports activities, distance vision is the primary need-for presbyopes too. Visual needs with sports progressives are different from those of general wear. The lenses are larger and the peripheral lens area is used more often and

more intensively. The whole lens surface of sports progressives is individually calculated, taking into account all data on the wearer and sports frame. The progressive is optimized point to point right out to the very edge of the lens, ensuring best acuity at all ranges. Tailor made progressive designs which takes into account the following factors are key to success in sports progressives:
- Subjects posture
- Frame position
- Amount of head tilt used for near vision
- Area of the lens used frequently.

Designing Prescription in Sports Progressive Lens

In designing the near addition for the high base curve sports sunglasses, the choice of addition is done on how the spectacle will be worn. If the spectacle will be worn for everyday use select the same add value and if the spectacle will be worn for sports, with occasional use at near, reduce the general wear add by 0.50 D. Reducing the add gives greater comfort in wear by reducing peripheral distortion and improved field of vision. The 0.50 D addition reduction represents the normally used sports near vision.

A general guideline for selecting the near add as under:
Sports spectacle tennis   2.00 D   if general wear addition is   2.50 D
Sports spectacle golf   0.75 D   if general wear addition is   2.50 D

■ SUMMARY

Sports lenses dispensing is a specialized part of ophthalmic optics. It is established that vision is critical to sporting performance. The art of dispensing is to maximize the visual information. While the eye care profession has traditionally been considered satisfying, secure and relatively paid, these advantages over recent years have not been encashed. The role of eye care practitioners is changing and as one door closes another opens. The market for sports lenses is expanding, lucrative and is now available.

Multiple Choice Questions (MCQs)

1. Which of the following optical error is caused because of the wrap configurations of sports frames?
    a. Prismatic error
    b. Oblique astigmatism
    c. Power error
    d. All of the above

2. Which of the following is not the principle advantage of high curve sports lenses?
    a. Enhanced peripheral vision
    b. Obeys the principle of 'Best Form Lenses'
    c. Barrier to dust and wind
    d. Decreased backside reflections

3. Which is the lens material of choice in sports lenses?
    a. Quartz
    b. CR 39
    c. Polycarbonate
    d. Toughened lenses

4. Which item is not associated with high base curve lenses?
    a. Increase peripheral awareness
    b. Increase dihedral angle
    c. Small size lens
    d. Recalculated lens power

5. Which of the following is true about polycarbonate lens material?
    a. It is linear thermoplastic polymer with an amorphous structure
    b. It is more impact resistant and lighter than CR 39
    c. The material is very soft in nature and hence prone to scratches
    d. All of the above

Answers

| 1. d | 2. b | 3. c | 4. c | 5. d |

Chapter 15

Specialty Lenses

ISEIKONIC LENSES

When there is higher difference of optical correction in the two eyes of an individual, it causes difference in size of the image and irregularities of peripheral distortion. The condition is commonly known as aniseikonia usually caused by anisometropia and can manifest with symptoms of headache, dizziness, disorientation, and excessive eye strain. An individual may find it difficult in attain binocular vision when the difference is more than 2.00D. Theoretically, these difficulties may be overcome by iseikonic lenses. Iseikonic lenses alter the size of the image but not the position of the retinal image.

Aniseikonia may also be induced by a pair of lenses of equal power which has been made up in different forms and thicknesses. The magnification or magnification created by a lens is the result of following factors:
- Lens power
- Vertex distance
- Base curve
- Centre thickness
- Refractive index of lens material.

The point to note is that the lens design is not intended to either remove magnification or to exactly match the magnification from both the lens. It is only necessary to decrease the magnification differences to the point where binocular vision is restored and patient's symptoms are overcome.

REGRESSIVE LENSES

Regressive lenses are extended near vision lenses designed to offer extended range of vision for intermediate and near vision to a presbyope. If a presbyope uses only near correction in the form of a single vision lens the artificial far point lies nearly at 40 cms in front of the lens and most objects lying on his desk top including the computer screen would lie in blur zone beyond the artificial far point and the subject would not have the clear view of those objects. The other solution is to use the regressive lenses. Such a lens would increase the extend the range of intermediate and near vision allowing him to see clearly all the objects lying at intermediate distance from the top portion of the lens and also near distance at 25 cms from the bottom portion of the lens. The range would adequately cover the most work area and would provide more useful intermediate distance field. It is very good option for presbyope who is an avid user of computer, pilots, surgeons and many others.

Progressive lenses, on the other hand are general purpose multifocal lenses providing the user a range of vision from infinity through intermediate zones down to the near point at about 25 cms from the lens. There is no distance viewing zone in regressive lenses and hence they are unsuitable for outdoor use. Regressive lenses are mostly dispensed as occupational lenses, satisfying the primary needs of user.

ADAPTIVE LENSES

Adaptive lenses are self-adjusting prescription lenses whose effective power can be altered by some mechanism. The power of the lens can be changed across the full lens surface or over the intended portion of the lens. They can be designed either as a lens system or a lens. There are different methods like fluid filled lenses, lenses whose refractive index can be changed by applying electric current or lenses with adjustable sliding components. There is a possibility of more innovations. Newer methods of designing adaptive lenses may be introduced with newer innovations in technology.

ANTI-FATIGUE LENS

Increased computer time, electronic games and other work and leisure modes have created for ergonomic products to reduce the various kinds of eye strain. Essilor's new anti-fatigue lens **(Fig. 15.1)** is the first single vision lens designed to reduce the eyestrain for the population of 20 to 45 years of age and has

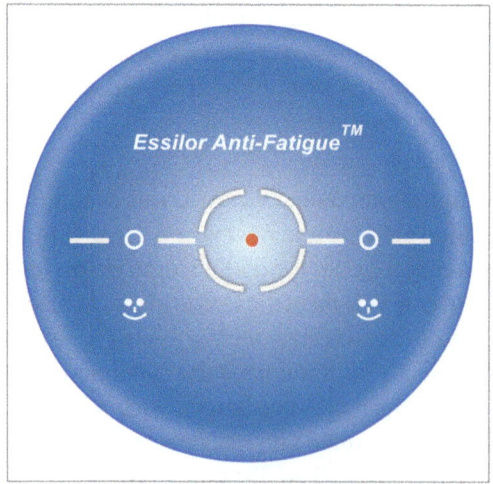

Fig. 15.1: Essilor's anti-fatigue lens

produced excellent results. Studies have shown that this age group has been identified as suffering extensively from visual fatigue. The lens is designed to relieve the symptoms of visual fatigue as headache, itchy eyes, reddening and blurred vision.

The lenses support the wearers accommodation efforts with an additional plus power at the bottom of the lens (+ 0.60 D). This provides a greater level of comfort for the wearer as the natural accommodation pattern is retained. At the same time Essilor's anti-fatigue lenses are not progressive lenses and hence have none of the limitations inherent in the design of progressive lenses. The lens design allows clear far vision and at the same time comfortable close and middle distance vision. They can be coated with anti-reflection coating also. The right and left lenses are symmetrical and the pupil centre has to be at the lens centre.

ATORIC LENSES

The rotationally symmetric aspheric lens provides excellent imaging properties for any lens prescription if it is in spherical. But in case of astigmatism prescription the two principal meridians require two different eccentricity **(Fig. 15.2)**. For example, in case the lens prescription is + 4.00/+ 2.00 × 90, the two principal meridians has + 4.00 D and + 6.00 D, which may need two different aspheric curves for the respective meridians. Such a surface is employed for the Zeiss Hypal series of lenses when dispensed for astigmatic prescription.

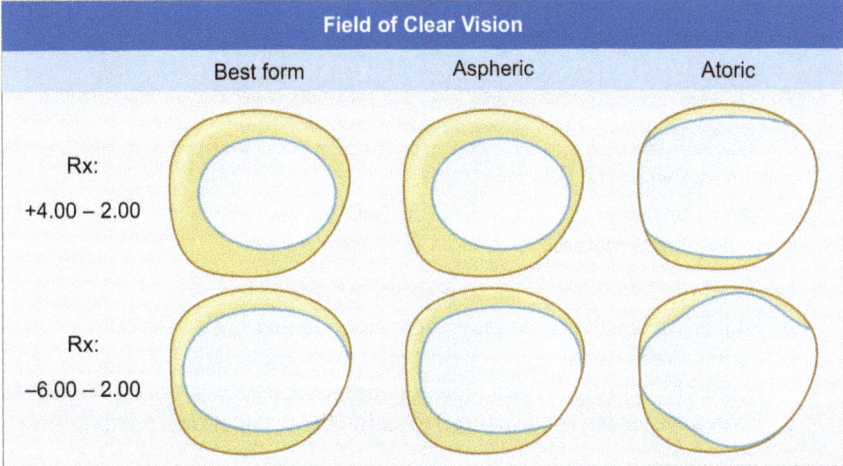

Fig. 15.2: Schematic representation of the field of clear vision with 3 different form of lenses. The white area in the frame represents the field of clear vision while the shaded area represents regions of reduced vision

Advances in lens design have provided the lens designers with the ability to produce surfaces that are even more complex than aspheric. Just as aspheric denotes a surface that departs from being completely spherical, atoric denotes a surface that departs from being an exact circular toric. In fact atoricity is an extension of aspheric lens design, allowing the lens designers to optimize both stigmatic and astigmatic lens. They provide a wider field of clear vision than the conventional best form lenses, especially for higher cylinder powers.

SUMMARY

The optical industry has certainly seen an avalanche of new developments in the ophthalmic lenses during last 10 years. The improvements have ranged from lens designs to lens coatings. The lens designers have really taken the challenge and looking ahead for newer lens materials with innovative properties so that one day they can fulfill their dream of making a lens which has:
- High refractive index
- Low dispersion
- Unbreakable and unscratchable
- Low density
- Aspheric in design
- Available in all multifocal forms
- Easy to tint and ARC
- Economical from the patients point of view
- More profitable from our point of view.

Multiple Choice Questions (MCQs)

1. Which of the following is considered as the power factor for the magnification produced by spectacle lenses?
    a. Vertex distance
    b. Base curve
    c. Index of lens material
    d. Center thickness

2. Which of the following is not true about regressive lenses?
    a. Regressive lenses are extended near vision lenses
    b. Regressive lenses are general purpose multifocal lenses
    c. Regressive lenses are unsuitable for outdoor use.
    d. Regressive lenses are dispensed to satisfy the occupational needs of user.

Answers

1. a   2. b

Bibliography

1. Bennett's Ophthalmic Prescription Work by KG Wakefield.
2. Ophthalmic Lenses and Dispensing, by Mo Jalie.
3. Ophthalmic Optics File by Essilor.
4. Optician's Guide by Ajay Kr Bhootra.
5. Practitioners Program Handbook, Published by Essilor for Practitioners Participating in Presbyopic Education Program in Asia.
6. Primary Care Optometry: A Clinical Manual by Theodore P Grosvenor.
7. Spectacle Lenses Theory and Practice, by Colin Fowler and Keziah Latham Petre.
8. Systems for Ophthalmic Dispensing, by Clifford W Brooks and Irvin M Borish.
9. The Product we rely on-Part 1 by Glynn Walsh.
10. Varylux Fitting Guide, Published by Varylux University.
11. The Principles of Ophthalmic Lenses by Prof. M Jalie.
12. Spectacle Lens Technology by DF Horne.
13. Optical Production Technology by DF Horne.
14. Website references:
    www.onlinecec.com
    www.mellesgriot.com
    www.visioncareproducts.com
    www.schott.com
    www.webwhirlers.com
    www.centershot.com
    www.saoa.co.za
    www.optics-online.com
    www.seikoeyewear.com
    www.firstvisionmedia.com
    www.laramyk.com
    www.essilorha.com

Index

Page numbers followed by *f* refer to figure, *fc* refer to flowchart, and *t* refer to table.

A

Abbe number 14
Abbe value 13
Aberration
    direction of 72
    types of 72
Achromatic lens system 68*f*
Age-related macular degeneration 93
Alkaline oxides 9
Anti-fatigue lens 234
Anti-fog coating 215
Anti-mist coating 216, 227
Anti-reflection coating 97, 104-106, 227
    advantages of 103
    principle of 98, 101*f*
    single layer 100
    technology for 105
Aphakic lens 116*f*
Aspheric fitting guide 118*f*
Aspheric lens 108, 110, 115
    checking lens power in 117
    design 110, 113*f*
    prism in 114
Aspheric surface
    anatomy of 112*f*
    measuring 114
Astigmatic aberration 160
Astigmatic lens 41, 45*f*
    axis direction of 43*f*
Astigmatism 168
Asymmetry design 161
Atoric lenses 235
Axial chromatic aberration 67*f*

B

Backward reflection 97
Barrel distortion 71
Base curve 222, 233
Base down prism 173*f*
Best form lens 25
Bifocal disk, solid 141*f*
Bifocal dispensing 142
Bifocal dividing line 131*f*
Bifocal lenses 120, 121, 134, 151
    B segment 128*f*
    curve top 128*f*
    design principle of 152*f*
    dispensing 143*fc*
    D-shaped 128
    E-style 128, 128*f*, 130*f*, 132*f*, 135*f*, 177*f*
        bi-prism 140*f*
    invisible 142
    optical characteristics of 130, 131*fc*
    popular shapes 126*fc*
    round segment 127*f*
    round shaped 127
    split 120*f*
    types of 121, 121*fc*
Bifocal segment shapes 126
Bifocal shapes 123*f*
Binocular vision 170*f*
Bi-prism bifocals 140
Blue light, spectrum of 94*f*
Broken laminated glass 202*f*

C

Cataract lens design 116*f*
Cellulose acetate 206
Cemented bifocal lens 125, 126*f*, 138
Chemical properties 18
Chemical resistance 207
Chromatic aberration 25, 66, 135
Chromium 80
Clear vision, continuous field of 154
Coating materials 105
    magnesium fluoride 105
    silicon oxides 105
    titanium 105
    zirconium 105
Coating on lens, layers of 213*f*
Color wheel 79*f*
Concave lens 34*f*, 36
    high index 15*f*
Constructive interference 98, 100*f*
Contour plots 164
Contrast enhancement 92

Conventional progressive addition lenses, limitation of 174
Convex lens 34f, 36
Convex surface 125f
Corneal reflection 98
Corning CPF lenses 94f
Corrected curve theory 25
Crown glass, conventional 78
Curvature of field 25, 70, 72
Curve variation factor 18
Cylinder error, concentration of 162f
Cylinder lens 41, 41f, 46, 48f
    detection of 46
    notation for 42
Cylindrical axes on protractor, orientation of 43f

D

Degree pantoscopic tilt 192f
Determine geometric center 223
Digital lens surfacing 28f
Diopter 5
Dioptric power, change of 223f
Dispensing sports lenses 222fc
Dispensing tips 104, 117
Distance optical center 157
Distance portion, optical center of 134f
Distance power 157
Distortion 25, 71, 72
Downward eye movement 171f
Dye tinting 84

E

Electrical properties 18
Electromagnetic spectrum 75, 75f
Equithin technique 172
Essilor's anti-fatigue lens 234f
Everyday frame 219f
Eye
    accommodation 155
    horizontal 170f
    protection 205f, 210
    rotation of 117
    turners, progressive designs for 187f

F

Face shields 205f, 210, 210f
Facial wrap 191
Far to near, clear vision from 154f

Field of clear vision 235f
Filters, code numbers for 211t
Flammability 207
Flint glass 11
Focimeters 175
Forms of curvature 4f
Frame
    depth of 189
    eye wire, tap on 145f
    front adjustment 191
    shape of 189
    size of 189
Franklin bifocal lenses 126
Franklin design 120f
Free-form lens designing 28
Fresnel prism 58, 58f
Frontal reflection 97
Fuchsia 229
Fused bifocal design 121f
Fused bifocal lens 121
    construction of 122f
    reading addition of 123

G

Geneva lens 37, 38f
Ghost images 103
Glass 201, 216
    chemically toughened 203
    high index 11
    laminated 201, 201f
    lens 104, 208f
    material 9
    photochromic lens 86
Goggles 209

H

Hard and soft design 161
Hard coating 213
Heat toughened glasses 201, 203f
High energy visible blue 93
High refractive index 236
High surface wetting angle 215f
Hydrophobic coating 214, 214f
    Water droplets on 215f

I

Infrared 77
Integral tints 82
Internal reflection 98

Invisible bifocal round shape 142*f*
Iseikonic lenses 233
Isocylinder contour plots 165
Isocylinder lines 165*f*
Isosphere contour plots 165

L

Laws of refraction 1
Lead oxide 11
Left eye progressive lens 156*f*
Lens
    aberrations 65, 66, 72, 72*t*
        types of 66*fc*
    adaptive 234
    blue
        cut 93
        light 93
    curvature 23*f*
    design
        astigmatism across 158*f*
        conventional 113*f*
        development 184
        progressive addition 169
    detecting prism in 62*f*
    dioptric power of 36, 222
    dispensing progressive addition 191
    edge of 221*f*
    filter 78
    first progressive addition 181*f*
    focal power of 5*fc*, 65
    form comparisons 24*f*
    form, categories of 24*f*
    housing, types of 209
    impact resistance 202*f*
    insert 146*f*
        marking on 193, 194*f*
    material 200, 207*f*
        refractive index of 233
    minus 35, 72*f*
    no line progressive 154*f*
    obeys Snell's law 34*f*
    optically compensated 227
    photochromatic 86*f*, 87*f*
    physiological progressive addition 182*f*
    polarized 88, 89*f*, 90, 229
    polycarbonate 12, 205, 205*f*
    power 233
        effect of thickness on 7
    pretinted 104
    regressive 233
    semi-finished 140*f*
    specialty 233
    surface curvature of 3
    surface power of 3
    surface tinting of 217
    thermally toughened 216*f*
    thickness 86
    tinting, methods of 82
    toughened 202*f*
    uncut 51*f*
Lensometer 46, 62
Lenticular lens 116*f*
Light
    reflection of 97, 98*f*
    sensitivity 92
    wave 99*f*
Liquid crystal display 91
Low dispersion 236
Low energy visible blue 93
Lower lid 146*f*
    edge of 146*f*

M

Magnification 137
Minkwitz rule 160
Minus cylinder 22*f*
Mirror coating 84, 217*f*
Multi-design progressive addition lens 182*f*
Multilayer anti-reflection coating 101

N

Near segment, placement of 144*f*
Near vision 151
Near vision area, location of 171
    vertical location of 171
Near visual point 134
Network formative oxides 10
Niobium 11
No visible segments 153
Normal glass lenses 202*f*

O

Oblique astigmatism 25
Oblique prism, angle of 60*f*
Ocular hazards 198*f*
Ocular tissues, radiant energy on 76
Off-axis astigmatism 69, 72

Ophthalmic lens 9, 13*f*, 19
   design 9, 19, 19*fc*
   material 9
   properties of 12
Optical center, position of 128*f*
Optical class 211*t*
Optical factors 23
Optical interference, principle of 98
Optical modulation, horizontal 181
Optical properties 13
Optician's lens measure 5
Optics, compromised 175
Ostwalt bending 26
Oxides 10

P

Pantoscopic tilt 191
Photochromatic lenses, dispensing tips for 88
Photochromatism, factors affecting 85
Photochromic glasses 10
Photochromic lenses 85, 86, 88, 104, 229
Pincushion distortion 71
Plano-convex cylindrical surface 44*f*
Plus cylinder 21*f*
Plus lenses 35
Polarized lenses, application of 90
Polaroid lens
   advantages of 90
   composing of 90*f*
   dispensing tips for 91
Polyvinyl alcohol 90
Polyvinyl chloride 58
Poor facial wrap 192*f*
Power progression profile 171, 164
Power variation, gradients of 168
Prentice rule 53
Presbyopia 230
   arrival of 120
Prescribing tints 91
Prism 50, 55
   and lens decentration 61
   at distance, different 57
   at near, differential 56, 57
   by decentration 55
   characteristics of 52
   compounding and resolving 58
   controlled bifocals 138, 141
   deviation produced by 52
   diagnostic use of 57
   dividing 54
   horizontal 211
   in optical lens, detection of 62
   orientation of 53, 53*f*, 54*f*
   prescribed 56
   therapeutic use of 58
   thinning 57, 172, 172*f*
   types of 55
   uses of 57
   vertical 211
   worked 56, 56*f*
Prismatic effect 133, 134
Progressive addition lens 149, 149*f*, 158*fc*, 163*fc*, 189, 189*f*, 190*f*
   advantages of 153
   anatomy of 157*f*
   design 160, 161*f*
      asymmetrical 162*f*
      symmetrical 162*f*
   evolution of 180
   markings 156, 175
   optical design 157
   surface 150*f*
Progressive lens 151, 155*f*, 156*f*, 170*f*
   design principle 153*f*
   power profile for 159*f*
   restoration of 176*f*
   shorter corridor 184
   skewed distortion in 174*f*
   sports 231
   surface, concept of 178*f*
   typical 150*f*, 151*f*
Pupil and lower rim of frame 190*f*
Pupillary distance 117
Pupillometer 193

Q

Quantum theory 98

R

Radiation 76
Rays, vergence of 36, 36*f*
Realistic color perception 91*f*
Reduced migraines 92
Refraction, sagittal planes of 111*f*
Refractive index 2, 14-16
Refractive status 188
Resin photochromic lens 87

S

Safety eye wears, types of materials for 200*fc*
Safety glasses, types of 201*fc*
Safety lens 198, 204
   testing
      parameters for 206*fc*
      procedure for 206
Sagometer 5, 5*f*
Scratch resistant hard coating 227
Segment lens, optical center of 134*f*
Sign convention 7, 7*f*
Single vision lens 151
   principle of 152*f*
Slumping glass blank 180*f*
Snell's law 3
Sodium 9
Sol-gel coating 105
Spectacle frame 209
   side shield 209*f*
Sphere 31*f*
Spherical aberration 25, 67, 68, 68*f*, 72
Spherical lens 31, 35*f*, 36, 37, 37*f*, 39, 69*f*
   basic forms of 33*f*
   concave 35*f*
   convex 35*f*
   detection of 37, 38*f*
Spherical surfaces 32
Sphero-cylinder lens, toroidal surface of 46*f*
Spherometer 5, 5*f*
Sport lenses 226
Sports frame 220*f*
   effects of 221*fc*
Sports lens 219, 230, 231
   colors in 227
   mirror coating in 229
Sputter coating 105
Standard axis notation 43*f*
Steeper lens 111*f*
Straight top D bifocal 128*f*
Strontium 11
Sulphur oxides 80
Sun lenses 104

T

Test ball speed 212
Thermal properties 17
Thin lens, vergence power of 34*f*
Tinted lens 75, 90
   types of 82*fc*
   varieties of 217*f*
Toric lens 41, 44
Toughening glass lenses 216
Transverse chromatic aberration 135
Trifocal lens 151
   design principle 153*f*
Two layer coating 103*f*

U

Ultraviolet 77
   light, components of 77*f*
   protection 226

V

Vacuum coating 105
Varilux panamic design 183
Vertex distance 193, 233
Visible spectrum 76, 76*f*
Vision
   comfortable intermediate 154
   print system 185*f*
Visual clarity, XYZ optics maintains 221*f*
Visual field, restricted 174
Visual needs 188
Vogel's formula 27, 27*t*

W

Wearer's face, adjusted frame on 144*f*
Wire gauze 206
Wollaston bending 26

Z

Zirconium 11

EU GSPR Authorised Reprsentative
Logos Europe, 9 rue Nicolas Poussin
1700, La Rochelle, France
Phone: +33 (0) 6 67 93 73 78
E-mail: contact@logoseurope.eu

www.ingramcontent.com/pod-product-compliance
Ingram Content Group UK Ltd.
Pitfield, Milton Keynes, MK11 3LW, UK
UKHW051846210426
5322IPUK00019B/274